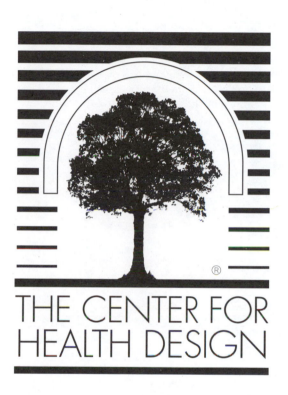

THE CENTER FOR
HEALTH DESIGN

# GARDENS IN HEALTHCARE FACILITIES: USES, THERAPEUTIC BENEFITS, AND DESIGN RECOMMENDATIONS

by Clare Cooper Marcus, MA, MCP
and Marni Barnes, MLA, LCSW
University of California at Berkeley

Published by: The Center for Health Design, Inc.

Publisher: Wayne Ruga, AIA, IIDA

Research Consultants:

Clare Cooper Marcus, MA, MCP
College of Environmental Design
University of California at Berkeley

Marni Barnes, MLA, LSCW
College of Environmental Design
University of California at Berkeley

Printer: Eusey Press

Design and Composition: Visual Communications

The Center for Health Design, Inc.
4550 Alhambra Way
Martinez, CA 94553-4406
United States of America
Tel: (510) 370-0345
Fax: (510) 228-4018
Email: CTR4HD@aol.com

Clare Cooper Marcus, MA, MCP
2721 Stuart Street
Berkeley, CA 94705
Tel: (510) 548-2904
Fax: (510) 643-6166

Marni Barnes, MLA, LCSW
Deva Landscaping
846 Boyce Street
Palo Alto, CA 94301
Tel: (415) 326-6866

First Printing November 1995
ISBN: 0-9638938-2-3
Printed in the United States of America

# THE CENTER FOR HEALTH DESIGN, INC.

**Vision**

To create a future where the built environment supports the highest level of human health, well-being, and achievement in all aspects of life and work.

**Mission**

To be a facilitator, integrator, and accelerator promoting the widespread development of health-enhancing environments, and the benefits that these bring to human health and well-being.

**Purpose**

To advance the quality of health design by:

- Supporting the needs and interests of its constituents.
- Serving as the internationally recognized source of educational programs.
- Supporting the development of research that will significantly advance the art and science of health design.
- Developing and promoting the application of design.
- Developing a worldwide network of supportive individuals, businesses, and allied organizations.
- Serving as a clearinghouse for resources, including: books, periodicals, articles, audio and videotapes, project data, facility tours, and product information.

# ACKNOWLEDGMENTS

WE WOULD LIKE to express our appreciation to the medical institutions that support and maintain the beautiful outdoor spaces observed during our research. Although many more people helped to point the way and grease the wheels during this study than we could mention here, some of the good souls are:

Alan Kinet, Bill Peters, and Gloria Rodriguez; San Francisco General Hospital;

Gail Uchiyama and Burton Presberg; Alta Bates Medical Center;

Irwin Fisch, Pat Mariani, Gabriel Escobar, Bob Eisenman, and Priscilla Minn; Kaiser Permanente Walnut Creek;

Karen Graham, Vicki Williams, and Francia DeAsis; California Pacific Medical Center;

Tom Piazza at the University of California, Berkeley, Survey Research Center, for his knowledge and advice;

The homeless and HIV-positive man who directed us to healing gardens in San Francisco;

Eileen Lemus, at Laguna Honda Hospital, for her knowledge and belief in innovative forms of therapy;

Finally, we are deeply indebted and offer our heartfelt thanks to The Center for Health Design and its Research Committee for sponsoring and supporting this study.

The Center for Health Design would like to acknowledge the following individuals and organizations for making this research project possible.

**Board of Directors**
Russell C. Coile Jr., MBA
Ann Dix
Kathryn E. Johnson
Roger K. Leib, AIA
Jain Malkin
Robin Orr, MPH
Derek Parker, FAIA, RIBA
Wayne Ruga, AIA, IIDA
Blair L. Sadler, J.D.
Roger S. Ulrich, Ph.D.

**Research Committee**
Janet R. Carpman, Ph.D.
Uriel Cohen, D.Arch
Syed V. Husain, FAIA
Debra J. Levin
Donald F. Lopez
M.P. MacDougall
Jain Malkin
Wayne Ruga, AIA, IIDA
Mardelle Shelpley, D.Arch
Karen Tetlow
Roger Ulrich, Ph.D.

**Sponsors**
This Research Report has been exclusively sponsored by: Armstrong World Industries, Inc.; Interface Flooring Systems, Inc.; JCM Group; and Jain Malkin

**Research Consultants**
Clare Cooper Marcus, MA, MCP
and Marni Barnes, MLA, LCSW
University of California at Berkeley

# TABLE OF CONTENTS

# 1. INTRODUCTION

THIS STUDY WAS conducted between January and August 1995, and its goal was to investigate the use and possible benefits of gardens in hospitals by evaluating a number of case studies. Its intent was not to propose theories of how or why certain environments are therapeutic, but to discover which specific elements and qualities in hospital gardens seem to be — in the users' eyes — most related to a change of mood.

This report consists of 12 parts: introduction; literature review; methods; brief historical overview of hospital gardens; a typology of health facility outdoor spaces; four case studies including user-responses; a set of design recommendations based on observations and interviews; and a conclusion.

Our consciousness regarding this topic was raised as we searched for case study sites. Hospital architects we contacted knew of few such examples. When we started to visit hospitals, we were surprised to find few that had outdoor spaces, and where we found some that did, the staff at the information desk frequently had no knowledge of the garden or its location. Thus, early on we sensed that this was a type of space that is considered unimportant in the contemporary medical center.

In all, we looked at 24 hospitals, almost all of them in Northern California. From this admittedly small sample we sensed that public hospitals are more aware of and supportive of gardens in their environment than are private hospitals. Two public hospitals in San Francisco — Laguna Honda and San Francisco General — are housed in 19th-century or early-20th-century pavilion-style buildings where open spaces between wings have been landscaped and developed as gardens. Both of these hospitals also run on low budgets, serving the needy, and seem to make use of everything at their disposal, including the outdoor space. Private hospitals seemed more concerned with cosmetic landscaping to enhance their image but not necessarily to fill the therapeutic needs of patients or staff.

As we conducted interviews, we became aware, too, of the pivotal importance of one person or a few people in creating and making known the benefits of gardens at specific facilities. The gardeners at San Francisco General created the Comfort Garden, a space that eventually became one of our case study sites. The director of the hospice at Laguna Honda Hospital was responsible for promoting the development of a garden in a formerly empty courtyard. (The timing of the installation of this garden precluded our selecting it as a case study.) Nurses at California Pacific Garden Campus were responsible for encouraging long-term care patients and their families to use the garden.

We are convinced that with more persuasive information as to their benefits, many more hospital administrators and medical staff would encourage the use of outdoor spaces for healing and stress reduction. We hope this report will be one tool in raising consciousness in this important area.

# 2. REVIEW OF RELEVANT RESEARCH

THE THEORETICAL UNDERPINNINGS of this project arise from four differing bodies of research on emotional response to the natural environment: (1) *viewing* natural scenes; (2) horticultural therapy, or *working* in a natural setting; (3) the experience of simply *being* in a natural wilderness; and (4) outdoor environments *chosen* by people as stress-reducing settings. There is a considerable range of research where subjects in a laboratory setting evaluate pictures of natural scenes after a stressful experience and are then tested for emotional and physiological recovery. These studies indicate that the presence of natural greenery in a scene has a high correlation with stress reduction (R. Ulrich, 1979, 1984, 1986; M. Honeyman, 1987; T. Hartig et al., 1990).

One significant study monitored hospital-patient recovery when looking out at vegetation as opposed to buildings, and found that those with a view to nature recovered more quickly (Ulrich, 1984). The second body of work reveals that participants in gardening activities report positive mood shifts. "Nature fascination," sensory joy, peacefulness, and tranquillity receive the highest ratings from the participants (R. Kaplan, 1973, 1983). Third, there is documentation of the influence of natural wilderness use, where people are asked to evaluate a place-experience. This research indicates that marked psychological benefits arise from being in a natural environment (Kaplan and Talbot, 1983; R. Kimball, 1983; A. Ewert,

1990). These psychological changes are often reflected in both short- and long-term changes in functioning and behavior (R. Greenway, 1990, 1993). A fourth area of research looks at where people go outdoors when emotionally upset. Two studies in which people were asked what kind of place they went to when feeling troubled, upset, or in grief revealed that natural settings were predominantly cited (Francis and Cooper Marcus, 1991, 1992). A further study related the process of emotional change to specific qualities of the outdoor environment (Barnes, 1994).

Though there are many studies evaluating the success of housing schemes, there are many fewer of healthcare facilities, and almost none of hospital gardens. The one exception of the latter is a Master of Landscape Architecture thesis by Robert Paine (University of California, Berkeley, 1984), which was re-written and summarized in the book *People Places* (Francis and Paine, 1990). Also important to mention is the tireless work by designer Vince Healy in promoting the inclusion of gardens in hospice facilities (Healy, unpublished).

Given the existing research on nature-as-healer and the garden/gardening experience, it is clear that the need for more documented, empirical research on gardens in healthcare facilities is critical. Case study evaluations of existing outdoor sites and their therapeutic uses need to be conducted to enable the development of appropriate and specific design recommendations.

# 3. METHODS

DESIGNED TO MEET the need for preliminary empirical data and applicable design recommendations, this research project undertook the documentation and analysis of exterior hospital gardens and their possible therapeutic benefits. For a number of reasons this study must be described as exploratory rather than definitive. First, there are no strictly comparable studies in the published literature, so there was no groundwork to draw on; and the necessity for breadth required by the discovery process precluded the exhaustive control of variables. Second, the time span of the project itself (January–August 1995) was very brief. Third, inordinate bureaucratic hurdles and wet and cold weather into May delayed the fieldwork. Hence, the bulk of the work — observations, interviews, site and statistical analysis — was carried out in a shorter time frame than was initially anticipated.

## Sites

The central focus of this research is on case studies of four hospitals in the San Francisco Bay area. Additionally, observations at 13 other hospitals in Northern California and at one in England were incorporated into the study. The three primary case study sites were San Francisco General Hospital in San Francisco (see Map 3–1); Alta Bates Medical Center in Berkeley (see Map 3–2); and Kaiser Permanente Medical Center in Walnut Creek (see Map 3–3). Extensive remodeling at California Pacific Medical Center Garden Campus in San Francisco — intended as our fourth

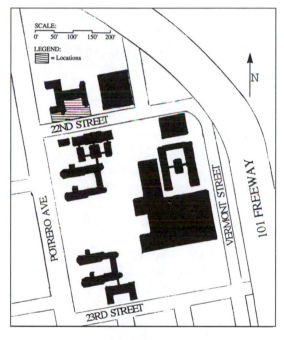

Map 3–1:
*The Comfort Garden, San Francisco General Hospital, Context Map*

case study — resulted in minimal use of the garden. It is reported as a descriptive rather than an evaluative case study (see Map 3–4).

Canvassing potential research sites revealed that there are actually very few healthcare facilities that have gardens that are utilized. This was surprising, especially in a part of the world where the climate could hardly be more conducive to outdoor activities. However, four sites were found that met the stated goal of attaining variation among the patient population types.

- San Francisco General Hospital's Comfort Garden encompasses the entry and lawn area outside an outpatient medical building (see Map 3–1).

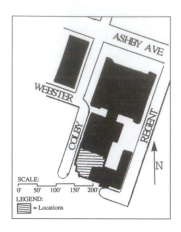

Map 3–2:
*The Roof Garden, Alta Bates Medical Center, Context Map*

Map 3–3:
*The Central Garden, Kaiser Permanente Walnut Creek, Context Map*

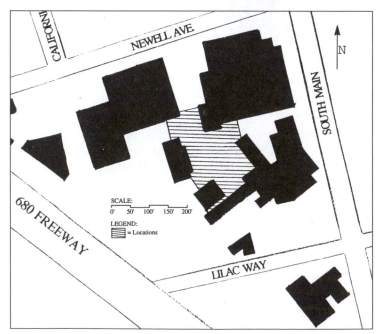

- The roof garden at Alta Bates Medical Center is adjacent to the maternity ward (see Map 3–2).
- Kaiser Permanente's central garden is bordered by both inpatient and outpatient facilities and by the cafeteria (see Map 3–3).
- California Pacific Medical Center's garden serves all of the long-term-care patients in residence there (see Map 3–4).

However, due to various hospital policies and construction projects, the results presented are not necessarily typical of facilities within their respective patient population types. (See discussions in the individual case study accounts.)

## Data Collection

In order to begin to understand the people-place transactions that occur in these types of environments, a multimethod approach was employed, incorporating visual analysis of the physical site, systematic nonintrusive behavioral observation, and information gathering through interviews.

The *visual physical analysis* of the site incorporated: (1) mapping of the physical design features; (2) circulation and orientation; (3) views into and out of the garden; (4) microcli-mates within the garden; (5) sensory qualities; (6) opportunities for social interaction; (7) opportunities for privacy; and (8) aesthetic and spatial elements.

The *behavioral observation* data focused on who used the space and what they used it for. This data revealed patterns of use that were analyzed to understand: (1) traffic flow; (2) user activities; (3) gender and age distributions; and (4) user type (patient, staff, visitor).

Each site was observed, and its uses recorded, for a total of eight hours: 11am–1pm and 1–3pm divided between two weekdays and two weekend days. Each session was divided into six 20-minute observation periods. To record the frequency of *uses*, if a given individual's stay in the garden spanned one of the transitions between the 20-minute observation periods, his or her activities were recorded more than once. (A person playing on the lawn for 25 minutes, for example, would be recorded as two user-observations.)

During the 32 hours of observations at all of the sites, a total of 2140 user-observations were recorded: 139 at Garden Campus, 154 at Alta Bates, 596 at San Francisco General, and 1251 at Kaiser Walnut Creek. The recordings at San Francisco General and Kaiser Walnut Creek underrepresent the number of people passing through the space, as the frequency of use exceeded the human limitations of accurate recording. The fluctuation of activity levels at these two sites created periods during which it was impossible for one researcher to record all of the activity. Note, however, that the people missed were the people moving through the space, and that this population was subsequently found to be less significant in this study than stationary users.

The user *interviews* explored what people liked about the space, what effects they felt it had on their psychological well-being, which qualities and characteristics of the garden they identified as contributing to their well-being, impediments to use of the garden, and recommended improvements to the garden. (See the questionnaire in the Appendix.)

Some questions, such as "How often do you come here?" were pre-coded into ordered categories: my first time; occasionally/sometimes; once or twice a week; every day; several times a day. Others were pre-coded according to information that had emerged from the systematic observations of use during behavior mapping. For instance, when asking "What do you generally do out here?" the interviewer read out 10 options and the interviewees were asked to indicate which activities applied to them, and to add any others not listed. However, the bulk of the questions were open-ended, allowing the interviewees to respond in their own words, and necessitating content analysis of responses during the analysis phase. These were questions such as "What do you like best about this place?" and "Do you feel any different after you've spent time in the garden?" Questions were asked in this way because there is no prior research that would suggest what an exhaustive range of responses might be.

When addressing people's feelings or change of mood, three approaches appear in the literature, each with a different level of reliability. The most accurate is monitoring physiological changes as an indicator of emotional shifts (galvanic skin response, blood pressure, heart rate, etc.). Self-reports are considered second in reliability, with the third, behavior observation, seldom used due to the extremely high level of interpretation required. This study drew upon self-reports because the need for a breadth of information and the fact that the cost and time limitations of monitoring physiological responses on hundreds of subjects precluded the use of this more reliable recording of mood change.

Although self-reports lead some subjects to answer in a way that they think is pleasing to the interviewer, the overall reliability of this method is nonetheless acceptable. Questions on other topics relied on self-report because it was the only way to access the information. For example, the only way to learn what people like best about a particular garden is to ask them.

The interview consisted of 25 questions and took approximately 15–20 minutes. The interviews were all conducted by the same person. At each hospital the interviewer made a continual circuit through the garden so that the entire site was canvassed. At the end of one interview, the next stationary person on the "route" was approached. Two limitations of this sampling procedure should be noted. The first was designed into the program, as it was anticipated that due to the length of the interview, approaching people who were moving through the space would be problematic. Thus, all of the interviews were conducted with stationary users and the responses of those passing through were not captured.

Another limitation was discovered during the course of the study. Although all individuals were approached, it was noted that individuals in some locations were more likely to refuse to participate than individuals in other locations. Those less likely to participate tended to be in the most secluded seating spots.

Twelve hours were devoted to interviewing at each site. It was hoped that 50 individuals could be interviewed in this time span. This was achieved at San Francisco General Hospital and Kaiser Walnut Creek. Slightly fewer (37) were interviewed at Alta Bates because of relatively light usage, and very few (7) were interviewed at Garden Campus because of building renovation and hospital downsizing during the course of the study. Although the drop in use at Garden Campus prohibits any statistical analysis at this site, it is reported with the case studies due to its value as a description of a long-term care facility.

## Analysis

The behavioral observation data were tabulated and prevalence estimates were established for each site and for the aggregate analysis of the combined sites. The open-ended narrative interview questions were analyzed for content clusters. For example, in analyzing the responses to what people liked best about the garden, the two researchers scanned the range of answers, then read each response and assigned it to an appropriate category. In analyzing the question about a change of mood, the selection of categories drew upon the work of Russell and Snodgrass (1987). Emotional responses were clustered into those that indicated a rise in energy level (felt rejuvenated, stronger) and those that indicated a drop in energy level (felt calmer, more relaxed).

Map 3–4:
*The Garden, California Pacific Medical Center Garden Campus, Context Map*

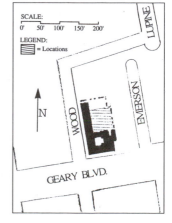

Three additional categories were developed in order to incorporate the full range of responses recorded: those that indicated a cognitive shift (find answers, think things through); those that indicated a spiritual or religious connection; and a residual category of those responses that were less definitive (felt better, pleased).

Descriptive results of the observations and interviews were presented both in the context of the individual case study and in the aggregate data analysis chapter. Comparative analyses were performed on the aggregate interview data, and noteworthy associations were reported. Several of the interview questions allowed for more than one response. This allowed for a discussion in terms of both the number of respondents and the number of responses. The associations made enable the comparative evaluation of the perceived beneficial effects of the garden on the user's psychological health, and the connections drawn by each, to the various relevant aspects of the garden. While rigorous statistical analyses were not appropriate, we believe these data do provide results that are an initial step in pursuing this line of inquiry.

Recommendations have been formulated for use in guiding the design of future gardens that are attached to healthcare facilities. These recommendations have been worded to be immediately usable by clients and professionals in the planning and creation of the next generation of therapeutic outdoor environments.

Overall, there are pros and cons to the methodology adopted. Among the advantages — given its exploratory nature — are the breadth of data gathered, the intersection of data from observation and interviews, the richness provided by open-ended questions, and the depth of researcher understanding via *in situ* data collection. Disadvantages include lack of experimental control of the interview environment, possible interviewee bias in self-reports, lack of a temporal perspective, absence of data from nonusers, and a relatively high degree of analytical interpretation (e.g., content analysis of open-ended questions).

# 4. HISTORICAL OVERVIEW OF THE PROVISION OF OUTDOOR GARDENS IN MEDICAL SETTINGS

WHILE THE MAIN focus of this report is to look at the use and meaning of outdoor gardens in contemporary hospitals, it is important to place this account in historical context. We are grateful to Sam Bass Warner Jr., who kindly allowed us to read and quote from his unpublished paper, "Restorative Gardens: Recovering Some Human Wisdom for Modern Design." This brief overview owes much to his work, as well as to a major published work by John D. Thompson and Grace Goldin, *The Hospital: A Social and Architectural History* (New Haven: Yale University Press, 1975).

The first flowering of restorative gardens in Europe occurred during the Middle Ages when hospitals and monasteries ministering to the sick, the insane, and the infirm often incorporated an arcaded courtyard where residents could find the degree of shelter, sun, or shade they desired in a human-scale, enclosed setting. St. Bernard (1090–1153) wrote of the intentions at his hospice in Clairvaux, France; his account of its sensory delights has some remarkable parallels with the self-reported benefits of gardens as conveyed to us by late-20th-century users in California.

Within this enclosure many and various trees ... make a veritable grove. ... The sick man sits upon the green lawn ... he is secure, hidden, shaded from the heat of the day...; for the comfort of his pain, all kinds of grass are fragrant in his nostrils. The lovely green of herb and tree nourishes his eyes. ... The choir of painted birds caresses his ears ... the earth breathes with fruit-fulness, and the invalid himself with eyes, ears, and nostrils, drinks in the delights of colors, songs, and perfumes. (Quoted in Warner, p. 80)

During the 14th and 15th centuries, a number of trends combined to render a decline in the monastic provision of medical care: Periodic plagues, crop failures, waves of migration into burgeoning cities overwhelmed the facilities that existed. According to Warner, with the decline of monasticism itself the significance of the meditative/restorative garden declined, and open spaces attached to hospitals became accidents of local architectural tradition, if they existed at all (Warner, pp. 7–8). The care of the sick fell upon civic and ecclesiastical authorities, and within the Roman Catholic tradition, one of the primary design incentives was to create long wards where the priest celebrating Mass could be viewed from every bed. The influential Ospedale Maggiore in Milan (1458), for example, was built in a cruciform plan like a church nave with windows so high that no one could see the formal gardens outside (Thompson and Goldin, p. 31).

Nevertheless, some hospitals did continue the courtyard tradition. Les Invalides in Paris (1671) incorporated a number of courts planted with rows of trees. The English hospital and prison reformer John Howard (1726–1790) described gardens for patients in hospitals in Marseilles, Pisa, Constantinople, Trieste, Vienna, and Florence. "In all these hospitals he admired the flow of fresh air, the chance for patients to see gardens through their windows and doorways and the opportunity for convalescent patients to walk in the gardens" (Warner, p. 18).

In the 17th and 18th centuries, the dual emergence of scientific medicine and Romanticism fortuitously combined to encourage the re-emergence of usable outdoor spaces in hospitals. The notion that infections were spread by noxious vapors spawned designs that paid special attention to hygiene, fresh air, and cross-ventilation. The so-called pavilion hospital became the predominant form throughout the 19th century. Two- and three-story buildings linked by a continuous colonnade and ventilated with large windows marked the design of the influential Royal Naval Hospital at Plymouth, England. The medieval Hotel Dieu in Paris was rebuilt with a series of 24-bed wards joined together at their ends by a service corridor, like the teeth of a comb (Warner, p. 23). These new designs incorporated outdoor spaces between the pavilion wards, while the rise of Romanticism prompted a reconsideration of the role of nature in bodily and spiritual restoration.

Recommendations for hospital garden design written by German horticultural theorist Christian Cay Lorenz Hirschfeld at the end of the 18th century uncannily foreshadow the findings of researchers such as Roger Ulrich at Texas A & M University, who documented in one study the healing benefits of a view onto vegetation for patients recovering from surgery (Ulrich, 1984).

> A hospital should lie open, not encased by high walls. The garden should be directly connected to the hospital, or even more so, surround it. Because a view from the window into blooming and happy scenes will invigorate the patient, also a nearby garden encourages patients to take a walk. ... The plantings, therefore, should wind along dry paths, which offer benches and chairs. ... A hospital garden should have everything to enjoy nature and to promote a healthy life. It should help forget weakness and worries, and encourage a positive outlook. ... The spaces between could have beautiful lawns and colorful flower beds. ... Noisy brooks could run through flowery fields, and happy waterfalls could reach your ear through shadowy bushes. Many plants with strengthening aromas could be grouped together. Many singing birds will be attracted by the shade, peace, and freedom. And their songs will rejoice many weak hearts.

The influential nurse and public health reformer Florence Nightingale (1820–1910) wrote with enthusiasm of these new hygienic hospital plans:

> Second only to fresh air ... I should be inclined to rank light in importance for the sick. Direct sunlight, not only daylight, is necessary for speedy recovery. ... I mention from experience, as quite perceptible in promoting recovery, the being able to see out of a window, instead of looking against a dead wall; the bright colors of flowers; the being able to read in bed by the light of the window close to the bed-head. It is generally said the effect is upon the mind. Perhaps so, but it is not less so upon the body on that account. (Quoted in Warner, p. 24.)

Good nursing practice by the end of the 19th century and in the first decades of the 20th century called for wheeling hospital beds out onto sun porches and roofs, and indeed in the treatment of tuberculosis, this fresh air and sunlight regimen was seen as the key to recovery. In the Catholic hospital St. Mary's, in San Francisco, photos in a corridor depict rows of patients in beds on the trellised roof garden. All that is now left of this space is a decaying segment of roof with a few flower boxes where staff retreat for a quick cigarette break.

The late 18th and early 19th centuries also saw radical reforms in the treatment of psychiatric patients and in the design of psychiatric hospitals. Psychological nurturance began to replace physical punishment as the core of treatment. New asylums were laid out with peripheral grounds and plantings to protect the patients from curious onlookers; landscape vistas were created to provide therapeutic experiences; and grounds maintenance, gardening, and farming became intrinsic components of the therapeutic regimen (Warner, pp. 30–37).

In the 20th century, understanding of germ theory, rapid advances in medical science, technical advances in high-rise construction and the use of elevators, and increasing demands for cost-effective efficiency led to the replacement of low-rise pavilion hospitals with multistory medical complexes. As Warner describes this trend:

In acute care hospitals, the design emphasis shifted towards saving steps for physicians and nurses, and away from attention to the environments the patients experienced. Gardens disappeared, balconies and roofs and solaria were abandoned, and landscaping turned into entrance beautification, tennis courts for the staff, and parking lots for employees and visitors. These trends which so captured the twentieth century American acute care hospitals spread, after World War II, by the processes of fashion to long term and chronic care facilities, to the hospitals of the Veterans Administration, to mental hospitals, and to nursing homes. The prestige of the big city teaching hospitals with their gardenless patient environments set the styles for all the others.

In one type of hospital — catering to long-term care of chronic illnesses — the garden was not lost. The profession of occupational therapy was established in the early decades of this century, extending a practice previously limited to psychiatric patients into the rehabilitation of patients with physical problems. After World War I, garden work entered the arena in rehabilitation hospitals; after World War II, horticultural therapy programs with special-purpose garden facilities began to be provided in hospitals for veterans, the elderly, and the mentally ill. With rising mortality rates from AIDS and cancer, the hospice facility has become more familiar in U.S. cities. These, too, have recognized the therapeutic effect of the garden. In the specialized facilities known as Ronald MacDonald Houses, for children with cancer and their families, a homelike environment and adjacent garden is the norm.

By the 1970s, general acute-care hospitals had come to resemble air-conditioned office buildings where the outdoor experience of most patients and staff was confined to the walk from the parking lot to the main entrance. A few had garden and courtyard spaces but almost never were these perceived as environ-ments that might contribute to the restoration of health. By the 1990s, insurance companies and hospital administrators competing in the burgeoning "healthcare industry" have generated hospitals that resemble hotels or even resorts, with elaborate entryway landscaping, plush foyers, art-filled corridors, and private rooms. The restaurant in Monterey Community Hospital with domed skylight, interior koi pool, and rattan furniture is so attractive that local business people go there for lunch.

Land costs and pressure from insurance companies to minimize hospital stays have largely worked against the provision of gardens in these new or refurbished medical complexes. "Landscaping" is often seen as a cosmetic extra — important to set the right image at the hospital entrance or in setback from adjacent streets, but rarely viewed as a significant adjunct to patient healing or as a setting for stress reduction for staff and visitors. Ironically, when suitable garden spaces do exist, inquiries at the information desk are often met with blank stares or an outright "No — we don't have a garden here." No hospital in this study provided any graphic directions to such a facility, or printed information for new patients. It seems as though the hospital garden in late-20th-century America has become an invisible and ignored amenity, and the possible restorative benefits lost in the world of high-tech machines, high-cost drugs, and increasing medical specialization.

The forgotten garden in today's medical arena might be thought of as analogous to the ignored psyche and spirit in the treatment of illness. The value of a garden and the role of the psyche in healing are both difficult to quantify or prove. But just as alternative or complementary medicine is beginning to re-examine the intricacies of the mind-body connection, so also are the design professions beginning to rediscover the therapeutic possibilities of sensitive garden design.

# 5. TYPOLOGY OF OUTDOOR SPACES PROVIDED IN HEALTHCARE FACILITIES

THIS SECTION PROVIDES an overview of the different types of outdoor spaces observed in hospitals visited during the study period (January–August 1995). With few exceptions, these were all in Northern California. A definition of each type of outdoor space is followed by one or two examples of actual places visited, observed, and critiqued in terms of their location and design. Each garden was visited for 30 to 60 minutes. Photographs were taken and a description of the setting and its apparent use was written *in situ*. All these visits were made on weekdays between 11 am and 2 pm, during warm weather. This proved to be most useful, as these observations expanded the understanding of hospital outdoor space and informed the kinds of design recommendations presented at the end of this report.

## 1. Landscaped Grounds

This type of open space consists of a landscaped area at grade that forms an outdoor area between buildings. It is often used as a walking route between buildings; a setting for eating or waiting; and as a space for ambulatory patients or those using wheelchairs. This is the most spacious type of outdoor area reported in this typology, and is sometimes described by users as "a park" or "a campus," and is often the hub of the hospital complex. One good example is at Kaiser Permanente Walnut Creek, described in detail in the case study section of this report. Another good example is described below.

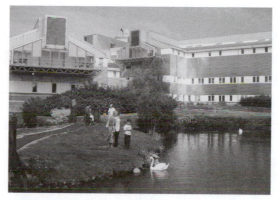

**Advantages**
- Can tie together a variety of buildings — by function, style, or age — into a campus-like setting
- Can serve a variety of users and activities

**Disadvantages**
- Maintenance may be costly

### St. Mary's Hospital, Newport, Isle of Wight, England

When a new hospital building was added to this 19th-century medical complex, the designers proposed a redesign of the central outdoor space. It is a spacious area and contains a lake filling a depression where building materials for the original Poor Law Hospital were quarried. The area around the lake was re-landscaped with lawns, paths, seating, new trees, two bridges, and two "pads" for the eventual location of gazebos. It is used by outpatients waiting for appointments; by staff walking between departments; by visitors or volunteers pushing wheelchair-bound patients; and by townspeople

Photo 5–1:
*A lake, landscaped grounds, and wildlife form a complete contrast to the hospital interior, provide interest, stimulate the senses, and draw patients, staff, and townspeople outdoors. A universally accessible loop path supports enjoyment by people with a range of abilities. Conservatories at the end of wards offer views to the lake. (St. Mary's Hospital, Newport, Isle of Wight, England)*

as a park where children are brought to feed the ducks and watch a family of swans who have taken up residence on the lake. It is a very attractive, naturalistic space and is as different from an interior hospital environment as any nearby space could be (see Photo 5–1). Obviously the provision of such a space is a rarity given the urban locations of most hospitals.

St. Mary's is able to incorporate this park-like setting because it is located on a spacious site on the edge of a small country town. The Kaiser Permanente facility at Walnut Creek is able to provide such a milieu (though much smaller than St. Mary's) because two "heritage oaks" in the center of its property are protected and a much-used and well-liked garden area was developed around these venerable trees.

## 2. Landscaped Setback

A landscaped setback is an area in front of the main entrance to a medical center, usually comprising lawns and trees. This is a space akin to the front yard of a house — to provide a buffer-separation between the building and the street. Also, like a house front yard, this space is not usually intended for use, but to provide a visually pleasing setting on approaching the entrance.

### Advantages
- May evoke a familiar, comforting image at a hospital entrance
- Provides offices or rooms at the front of building with some privacy

### Disadvantages
- While not usually intended for use, if this is the only outdoor space, its lack of seating, pathways, etc. may be frustrating for staff or visitors who want to use it

### Main Entry, Alta Bates Medical Center, Herrick Campus, Berkeley, California
The four-story stucco buildings of Alta Bates Herrick Campus face onto the busy street of Dwight Way, a few blocks from downtown Berkeley. A wide flight of brick steps with planters full of flowers leads up to the main entrance. On either side of the steps an area of lawn, facing south, about 25 feet deep, provides a setback for the building. It is punctuated by a

few trees and small flower beds. Larger street trees cast shade on parts of the lawn. There are no pathways, seats, litter containers, or other cues to suggest this might be used. This is the only green outdoor space at this facility, and might well be used if it were designed appropriately. Ironically, on the opposite side of this building is a paved plaza, over-provided with benches, and with none of the "green" and colorful image provided by this Dwight Way setback (see description on page 16).

## 3. The Front Porch

Most hospitals have some features at the main entrance that are analogous to the front porch of a house. These might include an overhang or porch roof, a turnaround for vehicle pickup and drop-off, seats, directional signs, a post box, phone, bus stop, and so on.

### Advantages
- Provides visual cue to main entrance
- Overhang may scale down size of building
- Sensitively located seating provides amenity for those waiting to be picked up or waiting for bus

### Disadvantages
- May be overused if it is only outdoor seating area provided
- May be under-used if main access to hospital is via parking under building

### Main Entry, Alta Bates Medical Center, Ashby Campus, Berkeley, California
The front porch seating at this medium-sized community hospital is sensitively located just to one side of the main entrance, where there is a lushly planted "eddy" space. People passing back and forth on the adjacent sidewalk, or walking in and out of the hospital, go by this small seating area, but do not go through it. Hence, people seated here — as if in an eddy off the mainstream — experience some degree of seclusion, yet can easily see if a taxi or a friend's car arrives. The seating is in the form of comfortable, wooden garden benches with backs. "No smoking" signs ensure that non-smokers will not be bothered by one of the frequent uses of spaces just outside of entrances to hospitals (and office buildings, campus buildings, etc.), that is, employees coming out for a quick smoke break.

**Main Entry, John Muir Medical Center, Walnut Creek, California**

A very large portico overhang clearly marks the main entrance to this medium-sized suburban hospital, as you approach it from one of the many surrounding parking lots. A semicircular roadway loops under the portico to allow drop-off and pickup at the front door. Two wooden park benches with backs are located on either side of the entrance, facing the roadway.

Since a public bus route serves this hospital, and people are being picked up by car or taxi, the location of the seating is appropriate. However, the entry faces west and summer temperatures are often in the high 90s. None of the seating areas has any shade; all look onto the glare of the adjacent road, sidewalk, and parking lots and receive the reflected heat from the building walls. Seating in the air-conditioned foyer is not close enough to the entrance to see when a bus or other vehicle is arriving. Attention to site planning, planting, or the creation of roofed shelters would have rendered this a more successful front porch.

## 4. Entry Garden

This is a landscaped area close to a hospital entrance that, unlike a "front porch," is a green space with a garden image, and unlike a "landscaped setback," is designed and detailed for use.

### Advantages
* Visible and accessible
* Makes positive use of part of site that might otherwise have been paved for parking
* Provides a pleasing image on entering hospital environment
* Allows use by ambulatory patients who want to see a little "action" near the main entrance

### Disadvantages
* Without sensitive planting, may be too exposed to nearby parking and entry road

**Main Entrance, Marin General Hospital, Greenbrae, California**

East of the main entrance to this medium-sized community hospital is a landscaped area with mature palms, live oaks, and eucalyptus, and paths zigzagging up to an upper parking lot. The trees screen out much of the hospital building; the views out from this area are of

hillsides covered with native trees and the more distant slopes of Mt. Tamalpais. It has a quiet, green, parklike feeling. Nine large palm trees border a small circular seating plaza. Around this are lawns, ivy-covered slopes, and a flower bed with every species neatly labeled. Two other benches, up-slope from the circle, offer a more sunny location. From the circle seating, nearby parking is barely visible, and traffic on a street that gives access to the hospital is heard only intermittently. Due to a steeply sloped site and the configuration of the buildings, this is the only outdoor space at Marin General, and it appears to serve its purpose well.

## 5. Courtyard

This is a space that forms the "core" of a building complex like the hole in a doughnut. Ideally, this should be immediately visible or apparent on entering the hospital so that visitors and patients know that it is there. When a cafeteria occupies one or more sides of the courtyard, it could function as an outdoor eating place. Trees for shade, flowers for color, a water feature for pleasing auditory relief, and movable seating are "basics" for such a space.

### Advantages
* Semi-private and secure; surrounded by hospital buildings
* Depending on location, may be easily viewed and accessed
* Shielded from wind; buildings likely to provide shade
* Likely to be of human scale

### Disadvantages
* Depending on its size and location, may create a "fishbowl" experience for those using it
* If too small to include adequate buffer planting, adjacent rooms may need to keep blinds drawn for privacy

**Cafeteria Courtyard, Novato Community Hospital, Novato, California**

This is a small, one-story community hospital in a residential district of a small town. The courtyard is immediately visible on entering the hospital. On one side is the main corridor with the Admitting/Registration Desk; on a second side is the cafeteria. The courtyard is accessed via sliding glass doors from both of these public and well-used spaces. The other two sides are administrative offices with windows that look into the courtyard; the windows usually have their blinds drawn.

The courtyard is small, approximately 40 x 40 feet. In one corner, the one sizable tree in the space shades a 9 x 9-foot pool with a central low fountain jet. The space is furnished with round tables shaded by umbrellas, lightweight movable chairs, and three garden benches near the pool. Color is provided by warm brick paving, some evergreen shrubs, a Japanese maple, and flower boxes of petunias and impatiens bordering the pool. The overall ambience is of a restful urban patio. The only aesthetically jarring elements are three large, humming vending machines against one wall and three newspaper vending machines. However, the former do offer a service for visitors and staff since the cafeteria is only open at certain times. Waiting for a relative who is in surgery; taking a coffee break; doing some paperwork away from the office; eating lunch with colleagues — this courtyard offers many users of this hospital a quiet outdoor respite (see Photo 11–5).

### Linnaeus Physik Garden, Santa Rosa Community Hospital, Santa Rosa, California

The Linnaeus Physik Garden at Santa Rosa Community Hospital is a good example of what can be done in a long, narrow, leftover space in the midst of a medical complex of old and new buildings. It is bounded on three sides by older, two-story hospital buildings, and on the fourth side by a half-open corridor providing access to administrative offices. It is not near the main hospital entrance, nor are there any directional signs indicating its location. However, on approaching the cafeteria, it is glimpsed through corridor windows.

The courtyard is approximately 40 feet wide and 120 feet long. The dominant aesthetic effect is provided by five, two-story-high maple trees arranged in a line along one long edge of the court. Under each is a raised planter of flowers bordered by a square bench. These provide seating places with a variety of views and varying degrees of shade. Between the

trees, and in a few other locations, are simple wooden picnic tables with movable benches, popular with groups of two or more who carry food out from the nearby cafeteria. During peak-use hours, some of these tables are in deep shade, some in dappled shade, and some in full sun — providing plenty of choice depending on people's tolerance for the sun. Since summers in Santa Rosa can be very hot, the provision of shade is essential. On the opposite, long side of the court are three sets of wooden garden seats with upholstered cushions — each set is a pair of chairs, with a small table between and an adjustable umbrella overhead. These are very popular and are in use both before and after the lunch-time users have left the picnic tables. Benches are often moved from one of the picnic tables so that users of these padded chairs — reading, eating, chatting, smoking — can sit with their feet up.

This courtyard has been planted with great sensitivity. The maples provide needed shade and — not incidentally — attract a lot of birds, whose songs and chirping provide soothing background sounds. Planters beneath the maples and along the edges of the court are filled with flowers; baskets of flowers hang from the roof of the half-open corridor. Two of the three entries to the courtyard are down flights of six steps; beside these are overflowing planters of star jasmine, so one's entrance into this space is marked by strong scent. Elsewhere in the plaza, star jasmine climbs the walls of the adjacent building so that all the upholstered seating areas are "perfumed."

This court was dedicated as the Linnaeus Physik Garden in 1986, when the hospital auxiliary installed six planters along the two long sides of space filled with medicinal herbs and plants from Central and South America, Europe, North America, Africa, India, and China.

The negative features of this space are the view at one narrow end onto dumpsters and storage bins, and the ever-present sound of air-conditioning units attached to adjacent windows that block out the sounds of a small corner fountain for all but those sitting quite close to it. The black asphalt surface of this court is not especially pleasing, particularly where the roots of maples have caused cracks and uneven segments. Warm brick paving would certainly have been aesthetically preferable.

### Medical Building Courtyards, Kaiser Permanente Medical Center, Vallejo, California

Three rectangular courtyards are bounded by the two-story buildings of a new outpatient facility. Three sides of each courtyard are corridors and waiting areas with floor-to-ceiling glass looking out to the greenery. The fourth side of each is occupied by offices and examination rooms with an ample boundary of trees separating these office windows from anyone seated or passing by in the courtyard. Some of the corridors are punctuated by cushioned window seats allowing patients waiting for appointments to have an even closer view to the outdoors. The staff at registration desks face out across the corridors, and they also have good views to the courtyard.

Although each courtyard is unique, they all have certain common elements: pathways of concrete pavers; geometrically shaped areas of lawn; low boxwood hedges; shrubs in very large terra cotta planters; long lines of trees (cherries and ornamental pears in one, Lombardy poplars in another); comfortable wooden garden benches and individual garden chairs with backs and armrests. Though these features are repeated, other elements are unique to each courtyard. One has a circle of poplar trees, a semicircular, seat-height wall feature, and is planted with a grass (clumping hard fescue) that need not be mowed and provides a lovely, wavy texture. Another has "beds" of black, river-eroded pebbles, a mounded lawn, and a specimen live oak tree. Two have wooden garden tables with dark green market umbrellas.

These all represent very successful courtyard spaces; they are highly visible, easily accessible, provide choices of seating, include high-quality details (seats, lighting, planters, etc.), and all provide a true garden experience. The only criticism would be that there are almost no flowers and there is limited seasonal color. Interviews at case study sites indicate that flowers and color are highly valued in gardens used for relaxation and stress-reduction. A specially sensitive aspect of planting was the choice of Lombardy poplar in three of the four courtyards. These trees move in a breeze and their leaves make a soothing, rustling sound. One oversight is a public address or beeper system that would allow people waiting for an appointment to spend time in the courtyard.

As attractive as these courtyards are, our impression is that they are quite underused. Were such spaces located in an inpatient facility, or near a cafeteria, we surmise that they would receive greater use and provide greater benefit.

### Children's Courtyard, Kaiser Permanente Medical Center, Vallejo, California

Half of this square, 45 x 45 feet courtyard is taken up with an attractive and well-used children's maze, constructed of four-foot-high wooden walls, topped by thick padding. Children waiting for pediatric appointments (or their siblings) try to find their way out of the maze, climb over its walls, chase each other around the perimeter paths, romp on the lawn (which makes up the other half of the court), or climb the sturdy live oak tree. They are easily visible to their parents in the waiting areas, but any noise that they make is not audible from inside. This is an excellent use of a small space, allowing children to let off steam in a hospital environment (see Photo 11–1).

## 6. Plaza

Plaza spaces in hospitals are outdoor areas, furnished for use, and predominantly hard-surfaced. They may include trees, shrubs, or flowers in planters, though the overall image is not of a green space, but of a paved urban plaza.

### Advantages
- Low plant maintenance and irrigation costs
- A small place can be designed for relatively heavy use
- Patients using wheelchairs, walkers, or crutches may be able to move easily in this space

### Disadvantages
- May have few of the qualities that people perceive as therapeutic in outdoor spaces — an overall green and/or colorful setting, a garden or oasis image
- May evoke the image of a shopping mall or corporate office plaza rather than a space for peaceful, stress-reducing, passive enjoyment

### Seating Plaza, Alta Bates Medical Center, Herrick Campus, Berkeley, California

This is an L-shaped seating plaza located outside the Oncology waiting area. The space can be entered from one of three doors in the Oncology Department, or via steps and ramp from Haste Street. It is about four feet above street level. Each "arm" of the "L" is approximately 75 feet long; one is 50 feet wide, and the other is 25 feet wide.

The feel of this space is of a highly designed, probably expensive, but rather cold urban plaza. There is a predominance of hard surfaces: travertine paving, now stained by water draining from the planters; 12 concrete, box-shaped tree planters; the windows and stucco walls of five-story buildings on three sides; the sloping glazed roof of a below-ground waiting area; steel benches; and a row of seven travertine slabs that tilt up into the plaza and down into the waiting area beneath. These latter, in particular, create a disturbing sense of imbalance in the space, and — unfortunately — are reminiscent of tombstones.

The planting in this space does nothing to offset the overall hard appearance. Twelve small Japanese maples are delicate and appropriate to this north-facing space but are completely overshadowed by the size of the adjacent building and the dominant hard-scape. Eight small pittosporum trees in planters between one arm of the plaza and Haste Street also do little to create a green setting.

The seating here is also unfortunate — six-foot-long maroon, steel benches placed between the maple trees in planters. Though they are reasonably comfortable to sit on (with backs and arms), their size suggests seating for large numbers of strangers at a bus terminal or shopping mall. Considering the stressful nature of waiting in an Oncology Department, it would have been more appropriate to provide short wooden benches or movable chairs, so that a person alone, or with a friend, could sit in a semi-private location. The eight benches could, theoretically, seat 32 people — an obvious over-provision in this location. Unfortunately, sitting alone in such a space evokes a lonely feeling, with so many empty benches in view.

## 7. Roof Terrace

Unlike a roof garden, which is located on top of a building or is usually open on all sides, a roof terrace is an accessible outdoor area that is bounded on one side by a building and often forms a long narrow "balcony" to that building.

The basics of such a space are plantings; a choice of seating types; a choice of seating locations with regard to privacy and sun/shade; and accessibility/visibility to potential users.

### Advantages
- Captures space that might otherwise go unused
- Potential for expansive views

### Disadvantages
- Depending on location, may be too windy, too hot, or too shaded

### Promenade, St. Mary's Hospital, San Francisco, California

This is an excellent example of a roof terrace. First, it is immediately visible through the large glazed lobby wall opposite the main doors into the hospital. Its outer edge is bounded by a long concrete planter filled with blue agapanthus and trailing rosemary. Just inside the terrace is a long walkway used for strolling and bounded by planters with seat-high concrete ledges. Off the walkway and forming the most prominent features of the terrace are two brick-paved seating clusters, bounded by planters filled with shrubs and flowers and shaded by pittosporum trees. The seating, with curved backs, is made of wood slats and is quite comfortable. It is arranged in right-angled clusters so that three or more people can sit together comfortably and converse.

The overall milieu is of a green and colorful urban garden with attractive, semi-private settings in which to sit, eat lunch, or talk with colleagues. The greenery can also be enjoyed by people working in offices looking out onto the terrace. The terrace seating is far enough away from the windows that the privacy of neither space is compromised (see Photo 11–3).

### Perimeter Terrace, Davies Medical Center, San Francisco, California

This is an unfortunate example of this type of open space. It wraps around the south and east sides of a central high-rise hospital building and is accessible by steps and a ramp adjacent

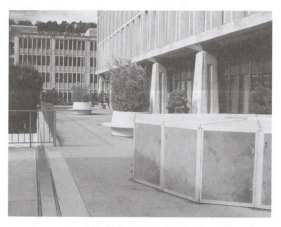

to the main entrance. Surfaced with cement, this is a stark, glaring space with almost nothing in it to tempt people to stay. There are a number of small, poorly maintained trees in concrete tubs, completely out of scale with the space, or with the size of the building looming above it. A few round concrete planters with seating ledges around them punctuate the space but offer little shade and provide seating that is uncomfortable.

So much more could have been made of this space, especially since on its east side it has a magnificent view of downtown San Francisco. The relative nonuse of the terrace is confirmed by the fact that the hospital administration has seen fit to place two large round bicycle storage containers in the space (see Photo 5–2).

## 8. Roof Garden

This is an area on top of a hospital building that is designed and landscaped for use by patients, staff, and visitors, and — in some cases — for viewing from offices and hospital units.

### Advantages
- Captures space that might otherwise be unused
- Private — unlikely that public would use it
- Potential for expansive views

### Disadvantages
- Exposed to elements: may be more windy than ground level, or enclosed courtyard.
- Depending on the growth and height of adjacent buildings, temperatures may be uncomfortable (too hot or too cold)

- Heating/air-conditioning units often vent on roofs, creating an intrusive mechanical sound
- Unless well signed, visitors and patients may not know of its existence

One example of a roof garden is described and analyzed in the case study section of this report (Alta Bates Medical Center).

## 9. Healing Garden*

This is a category that includes outdoor or indoor garden spaces in hospitals that are specifically designated as healing gardens by the administration and/or the designer.

### Advantages
- Users can expect that some thought has been given to creating an environment that is therapeutic
- Possibly disruptive activities, such as children playing or groups eating and laughing, will probably not be found in the space

### Disadvantages
- Depending on its size, location, and visibility, some people might feel self-conscious using such a garden
- If not designated as such, users may be confused as to its function

### Healing Garden, Oncology Deptartment, Marin General Hospital, Outpatient Medical Building, Greenbrae, California

This is a small (15 x 25 feet) garden in what otherwise might have been an unused space. On one side is a restricted waiting area for Oncology Radiation, with floor-to-ceiling glass so that even when not *in* the garden, it forms a pleasing green outlook. Two-story, cedar-shingled walls and the windows of several offices look out and down into this space, but the feeling while seated in it is not of being in a fishbowl because of very lush planting that seems to surround and enfold you. The plants — almost all shade-loving — are mostly species that have healing properties.

---

* Healing Gardens and Meditation Gardens are identified as separate categories within the garden typology. In general, meditation gardens could be considered a subset of healing gardens. A few hospitals studied had gardens that were specifically designated as one of these types. All of them had plaques identifying and dedicating the space.

Photo 5–2:
*A roof terrace near the main entrance to this urban medical complex is a disappointing example of outdoor hospital space. There is little color or greenery, the small trees are out of scale with the building, and the seating is uncomfortable and sociofugal, discouraging social interaction. Large bicycle storage lockers bisect the space and block a dramatic view of downtown San Francisco. Patient use from an adjacent day room is hampered by the lack of a wind-protected, transitional space. (Davies Medical Center, San Francisco, CA)*

The short paths leading to two seating places at either end are made of concrete stepping-stones set in moss. An unusual water feature — a grooved stone channeling a small stream down into a hollowed rock — provides a soothing sound. This is a very quiet and soothing space that makes wonderful use of a very small area in a sensitive way.

### The Healing Garden, Kaiser Permanente Medical Center, Roseville, California

This garden is part of a brand-new medical center that had only been open two months at the time of our visit (August 1995) and is specifically designated as a healing garden. It is rectangular in shape, approximately 75 x 120 feet in size. It is completely enclosed, on three sides by three-story buildings and on the fourth side by a 10-foot-high stucco wall shielding the garden from the parking lot beyond. The garden is entered from a — presently — little used corridor in the main Medical Building.

The entry door opens onto a small concrete plaza where seating will eventually be installed. The most prominent visual feature is a large set of planted terraces stepping up from a decomposed granite path to the highest point in the garden, the northeast corner, where a cork oak is planted on a gravel-based terrace. The three terraces are planted with forsythia, white roses, and orange-blossomed dwarf pomegranate. The slopes are planted with star jasmine and ivy, and heavily mulched with redwood bark. The flat, central section of the garden consists of a path looping around an area planted with dogwoods, blue turf lily (*Liriope muscari*), and dwarf periwinkle (*Vinca minor*), and punctuated with rocks.

The garden, of course, is still in its infancy; plants were being put in when we visited, and besides one litter container, no garden furniture had been installed, and no one was using it. Given the results of the case studies, this garden does not presently include many features or qualities that people reported as significant to them for relaxation. For example, the garden is not very green or lush, nor will it ever be, based on the plants selected. It has little visual variety, no auditory element, a limited range of colors, and the terraced section seems to have been designed for people to look down on from above, rather than as a setting to enjoy while in the garden.

In conclusion, the feeling is one of an interior, architectural space where plants are used for decoration, rather than a garden space that contrasts with the controlled and sterile interior medical environment. While an outdoor space design that extends the theme of a building to the outside may be appropriate in some settings (for example, a downtown office plaza), interviews at other hospital gardens indicate that it is the contrast between "building" and "garden" that people particularly respond to in a medical setting.

## 10. Meditation Garden

This is a small, very quiet, enclosed space specifically labeled with a plaque as a meditation garden by the administration and/or the designer.

### Advantages
- Provides a space for those in a hospital setting who want to be very quiet and contemplative
- By its name, precludes other, possibly distracting, activities (eating, smoking, etc.)

### Disadvantages
- If it is visible from indoor spaces, one might feel self-conscious, in a fishbowl. It is quite probable that only one person at a time might use such a space, depending on its size
- Given its designation, one might feel self-conscious about using it for other legitimate quiet activities that are not meditation (reading, writing)

### Meditation Garden, Marin General Hospital, Outpatient Medical Building, Greenbrae, California

This is a small (15 x 25 feet) court/garden space entirely enclosed by two-story cedar-shingled walls and windows of the building. The garden has low planting around its edges, an attractive stone wall, a fountain trickling into a bed of black pebbles off-center, and a path of decomposed granite looping around the fountain. There are four comfortable wooden benches, each long enough for two people, though they do not have backs.

The small size, greenery, and sound of falling water set the stage for what may serve at times as a contemplative space. It is close to the waiting area and is labeled on the entry door as a Meditation Garden. However, the windows of five offices open onto this garden and in warm weather, with windows open, the inevitable conversations and occasional laughter are intrusive. There is also something of a "fishbowl" feeling while seated in such a small space.

### Meditation Garden, El Camino Hospital, Mountain View, California

This new garden in a community hospital was donated by two couples — each of whom had lost a family member and had yearned for some place to go and sit quietly while in the hospital setting. The garden is approximately 40 x 40 feet and is enclosed by two-story buildings on 2½ sides. The entry is from a landscaped walkway through the half side that is open. The other end not bounded by buildings is enclosed by trees and shrubs screening the garden from lawns at the front of the hospital and a distant entry road.

The garden is dominated by four large weeping willows, which provide a green canopy, the sound of rustling leaves, and moving shadow patterns on the ground. Beneath the willows are shade-loving shrubs and ferns, scattered rocks, a dry streambed of pebbles, and a Japanese lantern.

A concrete pathway — wide and smooth enough for a wheelchair or gurney — leads from the garden entry to seating under a wooden-roofed gazebo in the center of the garden. Lighting in the gazebo and along the entry path permits use after dark — a thoughtful amenity in this area of hot summer nights. Windows from the Dialysis Unit on one side permit views out for the patients and staff inside. Reflecting glass in these windows creates an impression that the garden is larger than it is and eliminates the feeling of being in a fishbowl when in the garden. Two bird feeders hanging outside these windows encourage birds into the garden, which are then visible from inside and outside. There are also views into the garden from a staff lounge and a patient waiting room. Half-closed blinds in these windows permit someone sitting in the garden not to feel stared at.

Some of the drawbacks of this garden include: the low hum of an air-conditioning unit that competes with the pleasing sound of moving leaves; benches that have no backs or armrests and which form long right-angled arrangements, suggesting socializing rather than lone contemplation. There is one additional short metal bench with back and arms in which sits, incongruously, a green-metal, sculpted frog — a whimsical element more suited to a children's garden than to a place of meditation. The presence of an outdoor porch with tables and chairs off a staff recreation room at one end of the garden is also unfortunate, as the laughter and conversation of staff on breaks may conflict with the need for peace and quiet in the garden.

Overall, this is a soothing, quiet milieu that feels separate from the hospital. Though not far from the main hospital building and easily accessible, the garden's orientation off a path that is minimally used is a drawback that has impacted its use. Many staff are unaware of its existence, and patients or visitors are unlikely to find the garden on their own. The therapeutic benefits of such a space could have been enhanced with a greater variety of plant materials, engaging the eye to explore textures and colors while in the garden. Some movable garden chairs and paths to quiet, green corners would enable those who want to be completely alone and surrounded by nature to enjoy this space more fully.

## 11. Viewing Garden

With space and budget limitations, some hospitals incorporate a small garden that cannot be entered but can be viewed from inside the building.

**Advantages**
- Green space in a small area
- Can be viewed from comfortable indoor seating area — sheltered from rain; heated/air-conditioned
- Low maintenance costs

**Disadvantages**
- Greenery, flowers, etc. cannot be viewed up close or their fragrances enjoyed
- Fountain, birds — if present — cannot be heard

- Cannot walk, stroll, or sit in garden
- May be frustrating for some —"Look, but don't touch"

### Central Atrium, John Muir Medical Center, Walnut Creek, California

A small, square (approximately 32 x 32 feet) garden can be viewed through floor-to-ceiling windows from a large, plushly furnished foyer-atrium and from three adjacent corridors in this modern, suburban medical center. Flowers and ferns grow in square concrete planters of varied heights. There is a small fountain in the center and two 2-story-high trees. The garden was designed by — and is maintained by — a local garden club.

The garden provides a green outlook for people waiting in the foyer or passing by in the corridor. The trees are well selected, with delicate foliage that moves in even a slight breeze. The fountain, with a number of very thin falling jets, offers a view of water, but a fountain with more visible water would have been a better choice, considering that people cannot hear it. More lush, colorful, and varied planting would have made this a more attractive feature.

## 12. The Viewing/Walk-In Garden

This is a variation of the viewing garden in which a space that is predominantly (in terms of spatial extent and use) a garden to look out at from inside the hospital can also be entered and sat in by a very limited number of people. Such a space is usually viewed or entered from a waiting area or corridor.

### Advantages
- Provides a soothing green outlook for people waiting or passing by
- Provides a very quiet sitting place since few people are present
- The relative lack of use ensures that users of any adjacent offices or patient rooms will not feel that their privacy has been unduly intruded upon

### Disadvantages
- People sitting in the space may feel that they are in a "fishbowl," being stared at

### Internal Gardens, St. Mary's Hospital, Newport, England

Three small courtyard spaces seen through windows off the main ground-level corridor of this new community hospital could be characterized as viewing gardens. One has seating in it and is thus described in this section.

A door opens off the corridor and one steps into a space that is approximately 60 x 60 feet in size. Almost half the total area comprises tiled paving in a wavelike design, echoing a water theme used throughout the interior and landscape design of this hospital, located as it is on an island (Isle of Wight). Beyond the paving (as you view it on entering) is low shrubbery that acts as a buffer between the garden and the windows of offices/patient exam rooms on the other three sides of the square.

While the paving design is an attractive feature viewed from the corridor or from the two floors above, the detailing and furnishing of this space are less successful. There is one seating element comprising a circle of seats arranged in a sociofugal design (i.e., the seats face out, away from each other). This means that any more than two people entering the space together cannot easily converse while seated. Such a seating arrangement is suitable where strangers are sitting next to each other (e.g., a subway stop) but might be questioned where visitor-families or co-worker colleagues are the likely users. The absence of seating in several other half-moon-shaped paved areas that are bounded by shrubs and would have made very private seating spaces for one or two people curtails the use of this space. Also limiting the use of this garden is an inordinately high and awkward step up/step down entrance sequence. This, combined with the undulating paving (on a vertical scale), renders use by elderly or infirm people very difficult, if not impossible.

### Flower Gardens, Stanford University Medical Center, Stanford, California

At ground level in a new building complex of this large medical center and medical school, there are two walk-in/viewing gardens accessed from a major corridor at grade and viewed from three corridors, open stairways, and small waiting areas above. The gardens are very visible from inside through floor-to-ceiling glass. Beside one of these gardens, the corridor widens out to a spacious, tiled waiting area with comfortable leather armchairs. Thus, this garden can easily be enjoyed by numbers of people sitting inside.

The garden is roughly triangular in shape and is accessed by doors off the corridor-waiting area. The garden is approximately 115 feet long and 45 feet wide at its widest point. There are two seating clusters, each floored with concrete paving and furnished with five handsome wooden garden benches with backs and arms, plus a litter container. The two clusters at either end of the garden are linked by a narrow, winding concrete path that enables a brief walk through the garden. Around each cluster are a number of silver birch trees, three stories high. These provide some sense of enclosure to those seated, and the soothing sound of leaves rustling. At most times of the day, there is a choice of seating in the shade or in the sun. The birches also provide a green outlook for those in offices and patient rooms in the floor above the garden.

The planting in the gardens is exemplary: underplanting of shade-loving ferns, camellias, azaleas, and impatiens beneath the birches; massed plantings of blue agapanthus, pink and white roses, white and blue petunias, white cosmos, white and pink dahlias, pink penstemon, blue lobelia, and blue delphiniums. The effect is of a very colorful "cottage garden" with the birches in two corners and cherries in the third, acting as backdrop.

While one side (nearest the corridor) is obviously planned for use — seating clusters and pathway — the other two sides are faced by the windows of offices and patient rooms. The depth of the garden and the height and variety of planting ensure complete privacy for those inside. Although a distant air-conditioning unit can be heard, the overall experience in this garden is of being very remote from the hospital atmosphere, in a human-scale, secure, and enclosed setting, with the sound of moving leaves and views onto a wonderful variety of plants, flowers, leaves, shadows, and textures — a true oasis experience (see Photo 11–4).

Smoking is not permitted in either garden. Generally both were used by lone people reading and eating, groups of visitors talking, elderly patients in wheelchairs (with a companion) looking at the flowers and dozing, small children exploring in the shrubbery.

Having categorized, described, and critiqued a variety of types of hospital outdoor space that were briefly visited and observed, the next sections of this report comprise detailed case studies where systematic observation and user interviews provide a closer look at the therapeutic potential of outdoor gardens in hospital settings.

# 6. SAN FRANCISCO GENERAL HOSPITAL:
## *The Comfort Garden*

THE FIRST BUILDINGS designated as San Francisco General Hospital were erected on this site in 1872. Outbreaks of bubonic plague, the spread of tuberculosis, the earthquake of 1906, and the influenza epidemic of 1918 brought about severe overcrowding in this and many other San Francisco hospitals. Most of the present buildings were constructed during 1915–20, designed by city architect Newton Tharp in an Italianate style, laid out "with green lawns and bright flowering plants to add to the attractiveness of the structures." Early photographs depict lawns, shrubs, paths, and palm trees between the buildings, formally designed, but — apparently — with no seats or benches to encourage use by staff or patients.

The Comfort Garden is a small but well-used outdoor space in the sprawling contemporary "campus" of the hospital. It was established in June 1990 as a "living memorial" to hospital employees who had died. A name plaque in the garden, recording its inception, concludes with the words: "It is meant to be a place of solace where nature's beauty can bring you comfort."

## Physical Elements and Site Layout

The garden is located adjacent to Buildings 80 and 90 — imposing six-story brick buildings with many operable windows looking out over the outdoor space. These buildings house a variety of clinics, including those for TB, HIV, methadone maintenance, Family Health,

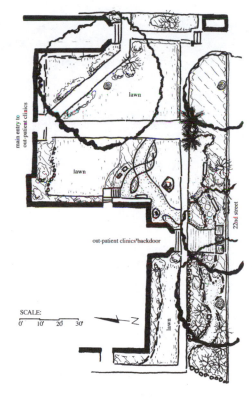

Map 6–1:
*Comfort Garden,
Illustrative Plan*

and Child Abuse. All of these are *out*patient clinics; none of the buildings adjacent to the Comfort Garden contains inpatient beds. The garden is bounded on two sides by these buildings and on the other two sides by fences that separate it from 22nd Street and a parking lot.

The feeling of this residential-scale garden is of a green and colorful retreat (see Map 6–1). Three very large trees — one cedar and two Monterey pines — are almost as tall as the buildings. Five lawn areas are bounded by concrete paths and flower beds. Most of the paths are designed for easy, direct pedestrian

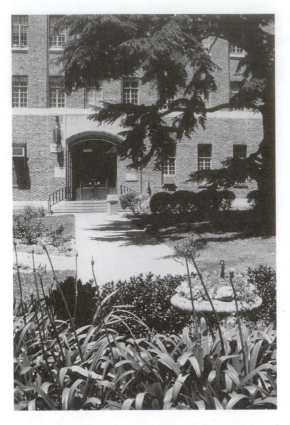

Photo 6–1:
*Main entry path
to Building 90 —
the busiest route
through the gar-
den on weekdays*

Richards, is entitled "Companion Place — a complement to the Comfort Garden." It comprises a curvilinear path bounded by granite blocks and surfaced with decomposed granite; five large granite blocks that function as casual seating; and two granite-bordered flower beds planted more formally than the rest of the garden, with African marigolds and lobelia.

Within and beside the informal flower border that runs the length of the garden on its southwest side, there are a variety of places to sit (see Map 6–2). Two wooden benches with backs and arms are a perfect size for two people to occupy for a private conversation, or for one person to "claim" by sitting lengthwise with feet up. These are ideal choices for this garden considering its size and image. Being of small scale, and of more delicate construction, they are clearly *garden* benches rather than park benches (see Photo 6–3). Under one of the large pine trees the gardeners have built a simple wooden platform. This enables two to four people to sit, backs against the tree, their feet up, their lunch or coffee or book beside them. It is pleasantly informal, flexible in use, and far enough away from a path to be relatively private.

Also providing informal seating are a row of large tree stumps forming the border of a

movement (see Photo 6–1), but one made of decomposed granite and another formed with "steppingstone" blocks of wood are clearly designed for more casual strolling. The latter winds through a lushly planted garden bed where shrubs and flowers can be viewed at close quarters (see Photo 6–2).

Photo 6–2:
*Strolling path and
secluded bench in
the long flower
border*

This is clearly a garden that has been created — and is maintained — with love and care: Tree stumps have been arranged to border flower beds; an arbor has been created out of thin branches pruned from nearby trees; rocks have been placed among the flowers; annuals are planted out in colorful displays. There are no weeds, nor is there any litter; yet the garden has a casual rather than a manicured appearance.

When this study was conducted — May–June 1995 — there were no fewer than 35 different species of plants and shrubs in bloom. No wonder one of our interviewees, when asked what she would like to see changed, asked for plant labels.

While most of the Comfort Garden has a casual, "country cottage" garden image, a portion of it was changed in 1994 to add a more formal sculptural element. This area, by Peter

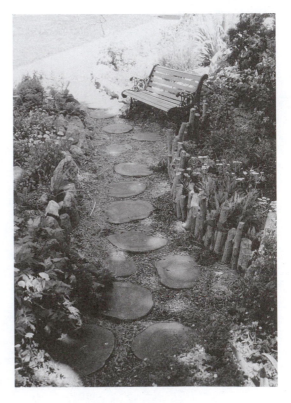

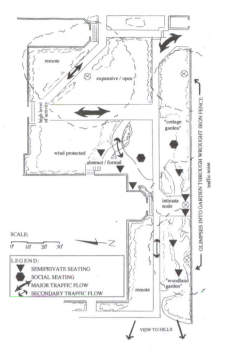

Map 6–2:
*Comfort Garden,
Experiential
Analysis*

and colorful planting, particularly in contrast to adjacent streets and tall brick buildings; two, the relatively enclosed feeling when in the garden. On one long side, it is bounded by the four- to six-story wings of Buildings 80 and 90. On the opposite long side, its immediate boundary is a 10-foot iron fence, densely covered in parts by a flowering vine. Beyond this, on the other side of 22nd Street, the space is visually bounded by the three and four stories of another brick hospital wing.

The top southeast end of the garden is defined by a low laurel hedge, but is visually bounded by the concrete end wall of the hospital heating plant viewed through trees, and by a large modern addition to the hospital (see Photo 6–4). At the downhill, narrow northwest end of the garden, an iron fence forms an edge along Portrero Avenue, but the two-story row houses across the street and more distant hills of Twin Peaks form a more effective visual boundary. These enclosing elements, together with its modest size, effectively complement the rich planting to create an oasislike effect. At its widest, the garden is just under 100 feet, while it is approximately 160 feet long. The scale of this space evokes much

portion of the long flower border. Though right next to a path, this is one of the least-used walkways in the garden, and therefore there is some degree of privacy.

## Microclimate and Ambience

On a sunny day in spring and summer during the peak-use hours (11 a.m. – 2 p.m.), approximately 85 percent of the garden is in the sun. However, this part of San Francisco is quite frequently breezy, if not windy. On a sunny and breezy day, the comfort difference between sitting in the sun and sitting in the shade is quite marked. Fortunately, both garden benches and all the granite seating blocks are in the sun almost all day. The wooden-platform seating, underneath a large Monterey pine, is in shade most of the time. Thus, only on the hottest and calmest days is this a comfortable place to rest.

A small number of those we interviewed complained that the garden is "too noisy." Indeed, there is a fair degree of background noise in this setting: cars and buses driving past on Portrero Avenue; cars accelerating uphill on 22nd Street; and the sounds from a large air-conditioning unit on an adjacent building.

When asked to describe the garden, some referred to it as "an oasis." We suspect that this image is evoked by two things: one, the lush

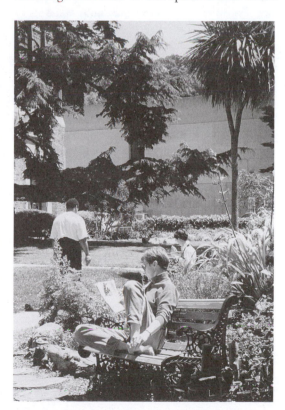

Photo 6–3:
*Garden benches
are an ideal size for
one individual to
"claim" and to
provide some privacy for reading
or eating.*

Map 6–3:
*Comfort Garden,
Users Passing
Through*

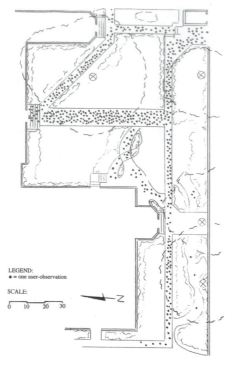

LEGEND:
• = one user-observation

SCALE:
0   10   20   30

N

more of a garden feeling than, say, the experience of a park (see Photo 6–5).

## Garden Use

A central path in the garden leads to one of the main entrances to this wing of the hospital (see Photo 6–1). Not surprisingly, walking to and from this and three lesser-used doorways comprises four-fifths of the use of this space (see Map 6–3). While only one-fifth of the total of 297 observed users comprised people standing, sitting, or lying down, the significance of these users should not be underestimated: They stayed much longer than the walkers-through, and they seemed to *enjoy* the garden more — pointing out plants, smelling the roses, lying on the lawn on warm days, eating lunch, chatting with friends or colleagues (see Photo 6–3).

The typical stationary users were staff members who came out to stand or sit while smoking; staff members who came out alone or in pairs to enjoy eating a brown-bag lunch; visitors or patients who sat for a while, sometimes smoking or drinking, or who lay dozing on the lawn (see Map 6–4). It was not uncommon at lunch time to see staff members come out and look around for a vacant bench and find them all full. Two-fifths of those interviewed reported

Photo 6–4:
*Visual boundary at
top end of garden
is created by the
hospital heating
plant, new hospital
building, and old
brick wing.*

staying in the garden for 30 minutes or more when they came out. There was no significant difference between the use of the garden and the length of time people stayed between staff and outpatients or visitors.

## Interviews with Users of the Comfort Garden

In all, a total of 50 people who were spending time in the garden were interviewed. Of these, 31 were men and 19 were women; 24 were staff and employees, 20 were outpatients, 5 were visitors, and 1 was an inpatient. When asked how *often* they used the garden, close to half said "up to twice a week." A substantial number use the garden at least once a day (see Figure 1). Not only did a considerable number use the garden frequently, but also almost half of the users reported that on some visits they stayed 30 minutes or longer.

We showed interviewees a list of possible activities in the garden and asked them to check as many as were relevant. Every person interviewed said that he or she came to the garden to relax. Three-quarters of the users reported that they also came into the garden to eat. More than half said that they came here to talk, stroll along the paths, partake of their own "outdoor therapy," or to wait.

Two-thirds came into the garden alone, and just under a third came with one other person. This confirms that the scale of seating provided appears to accommodate the needs of many users — short benches and granite blocks that can be "claimed" by a person sitting alone or can comfortably accommodate two friends.

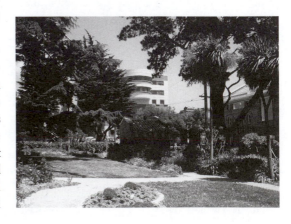

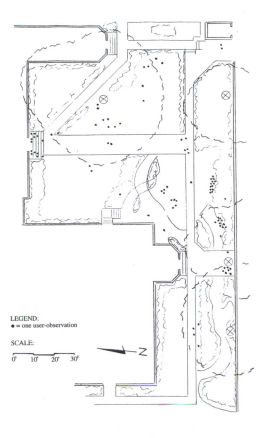

LEGEND:
● = one user-observation

SCALE:
0'   10'   20'   30'

N

Map 6–4:
*Comfort Garden,
Stationary Users*

Clearly, for most people who spent time in it, the garden facilitated a change in mood that was positive. They left after a medical appointment, or returned to work in the hospital, feeling less stressed, refreshed, more content.

For example, a middle-aged male outpatient who comes to the hospital once or twice a week reported:

> It's a good escape from what they put me through. I come out here between appointments. I enjoy the air, the feel of the sun, the privacy — everyone inside knows me; I don't know anyone out here. It gives me the strength to deal with things. I feel much calmer, less stressed.

A young female employee reported:

> My level of stress goes way down. I'm a lot more relaxed; I go back to work refreshed. ... It feels like something is alive here in the middle of a city that seems dead.

## FIGURE 1

### *Frequency of Use Reported by Interviewees*

First time here 14%

Up to twice a week 46%

Every day and more 40%

A middle-aged male outpatient who comes to the garden every day to sit, relax, stroll, talk, eat, and meditate loves the solitude and

## What Happens to People in the Comfort Garden

When asked, "Do you feel any different after you've spent time in the garden?," half said that they felt calmer, more relaxed, less stressed. These comments were made by both staff and outpatients (see Table 6–1). A significant number reported feeling "better, stronger, more positive." These respondents were mostly outpatients.

## TABLE 6–1

### *Percent of Respondents Reporting Various Types of Mood Changes*

|  | Percent |
|---|---|
| Calmer, contented, sleepy, more relaxed, less stressed | 68 |
| Better, more positive, pleased | 26 |
| Refreshed, stronger | 16 |
| Helps me think through problems | 10 |
| Moves me, a religious connection | 6 |
| Escape from work | 4 |
| No difference in mood | 4 |

(Number of respondents: 50)

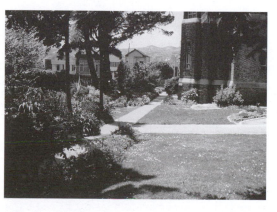

Photo 6–5:
*This long path leads up into the garden from the bus stop and a small employee parking lot. Note the visual boundary created by the houses on Potrero Boulevard and by distant outline of Twin Peaks.*

the colors and leaves the garden feeling "more relaxed ... it's very peaceful, an oasis ... sometimes I come here all wound up and then I feel relaxed."

A female visitor who comes once a week and waits for a friend while he's at an appointment remarked:

> It's pretty, it's relaxing ... visual beauty lifts my spirits. I feel that any plant life has a big effect on people. ... I've come out here and picked flowers for a friend who was dying because I didn't have any money, and it made her feel better.

## What Users Liked Best About the Garden

By relating how they would describe the garden to someone who had never been here, the interviewees revealed what was significant to them about its design and image. One middle-aged male patient who relaxes, eats, or drinks in the garden once or twice a week described it as "... absolutely beautiful ... it's like a rainbow on a beautiful day, with a beautiful woman. How do you describe color to a blind man?" Many referred to it as "an oasis in a sterile setting," or "a little bit of heaven," "a paradise." People seemed to appreciate especially its well-tended yet casual atmosphere; several referred to it as being "like an English country garden," or "like a garden in someone's home."

These very positive responses to the garden were further confirmed when people were asked: "What do you like best about this place?"

TABLE 6–2

*Percent of Respondents Who Named These Qualities as What They Liked Best*

|  | Percent |
| --- | --- |
| Aesthetic attractiveness and design | 92 |
| Flowers, plants, trees | 74 |
| Privacy, quiet, comfort | 60 |
| Open air, sun, seasonal change, birds, butterflies | 24 |
| Human companionship | 10 |
| Memories of friends who have died | 4 |

(Number of respondents: 50)

The flowery, lush, and oasislike qualities were again emphasized, but so too were the feelings and activities this place supported. Two outpatients remarked: "It's a place where you can come and think without a whole lot of people around"; "I feel more comfortable when I'm around other people who are ill or recovering — they're in the same position as me." A female employee who works in a child abuse clinic brings children out to the garden: "It relaxes them, if they had a traumatic experience. I point out the flowers, let them play." A male employee who works in HIV research likes the colorfulness, the variety, and "the fact that there are plants in memory of some of my co-workers who have died. A lot of the patients I see have died. Sometimes it seems like a place they'd come back to if they're coming around to visit." Several employees and outpatients had tears in their eyes as they described the memorial or spiritual significance of the garden.

## Changes and Modifications Desired in the Garden

When asked if there were anything they would like to see changed or added to the garden, the most frequent response was — "Nothing!" or "It's changing all the time — flowers, the seasons, what the gardeners do."

TABLE 6–3

*Percent of Respondents Who Desired These Changes*

|  | Percent |
| --- | --- |
| Change nothing; it is changing | 36 |
| Practical changes: more seats, tables, ashtrays, trash cans | 32 |
| More flowers, trees, shade | 22 |
| Make larger and more private; add kids' play area, cut out noise | 20 |
| Ban dogs and smokers; improve maintenance | 14 |
| Aesthetic changes: add arbor, water feature, wrought iron, more paths, label plants | 12 |
| Protect/enhance the personal meaning | 4 |

(Number of respondents: 50)

There was a desire for more places to sit and for picnic tables; also for things to improve maintenance such as additional trash cans, banning dogs and smokers. The latter — if enforced — would certainly decrease use since many users were observed smoking while standing or sitting in the garden or strolling through. Recent bans on smoking in public buildings in California have meant that public outdoor space is increasingly used for this activity.

While some desired improvements were voiced in response to this question, the overall tone of those we spoke with was of strongly felt appreciation and love for this place, and for the care of the gardeners who created and maintain it.

Two comments regarding changes are particularly pertinent to the kinds of outpatients visiting clinics in the adjacent buildings. A patient with AIDS, beginning to lose weight, remarked on the need for *padded* seating. Patients on methadone maintenance used the garden to "space out" and wanted nothing changed. "Where else would I go?" one asked. It was clear that some users were on the fringe of society, if not actually homeless; for them, especially, the garden was a nurturing setting where they felt comfortable and at home.

## Weekend and Weekday Use

There is a very marked difference in the use of this garden between weekdays and weekends. On weekdays, the clinics are open and staff are on duty. There is barely a moment between 10 AM and 5 PM when people (often many at a time) are not streaming in and out of the adjacent buildings. During the middle hours of the day, as noted, many use it for eating lunch, taking a break, lying in the sun, etc.

On weekends, however, clinics are closed. Almost no one enters or leaves the buildings. The few who walk through tend to follow the long path running from one end to the other, and to use the space as a neighborhood park. A couple with a small boy walk slowly through, stopping frequently to look at the flowers; the boy balances on a log-wall, holding his father's hand. A little girl on a bike rides down the path calling out to her father, who walks behind carrying a baseball bat and mitt and leading a dog. A young man walks two small dogs. Three youths on mountain bikes bump along the "rustic" path made of logs and chips. It appears as though all these are local residents, enjoying the garden as a neighborhood outdoor space.

## Conclusion

The Comfort Garden at San Francisco General Hospital is a remarkable, well-loved oasis that brings joy, contentment, and peace to visitors and outpatients visiting clinics in adjacent buildings, and to medical and administrative staff who work nearby. Its informal design, lush plant growth, and loving maintenance by the gardeners who created this oasislike setting are clearly highly appreciated by all kinds of users, by those who pass through as well as those who spend more time there. Of the few changes requested, some — more seats, tables, and so on — could conceivably be effected, while others — less noise, larger size, etc. — are of a more structural nature. While those we talked with had varying abilities to articulate what effect the garden seems to have upon their feelings, there seems no doubt that all but a few were affected very positively. In various ways, and in differing degrees, this does indeed appear to be a "healing garden."

# 7. CASE STUDY: ALTA BATES MEDICAL CENTER, BERKELEY, CALIFORNIA:
## *The Roof Garden*

THIS IS A complex of three- to six-story buildings set in a neighborhood of single-family homes, apartments, and medical office buildings in South Berkeley. It is named for Alta Alice Miner Bates, who first settled in Berkeley in 1904, and nursed patients in her parents' home as there was no hospital in the community. In 1905, at the request of local physicians, and with plans drawn up by her contractor-father, she built an eight-bed nursing facility and school for nurses on Dwight Way, called Alta Bates Sanitarium. In 1908, due to population growth in Berkeley after the 1906 earthquake, the facility moved to large three-story buildings at its present site on Webster Street.

In 1928, its name was changed to Alta Bates Hospital and six-story buildings were added. Care was taken through setbacks and landscaping to ensure that the buildings blended into the residential neighborhood. This concern extended into the 1980s, when the old buildings were replaced by modern facilities and set back from Ashby Avenue behind lawns and trees. The roof garden — dedicated to the Alta Bates Volunteer Auxiliary — was opened on the third floor of a new building in 1983. It is accessed from elevators 9 and 10, which are approached via a long corridor leading south from the main lobby. There is no indication or sign in the main lobby directing people to it, and inquiries at the information desk suggest that the volunteers who work there do not know of its existence or assume it is not for public use. Upon finding one's way to remote elevators 9 and 10, only an enigmatic "R" button in the elevator indicates its presence.

## Physical Elements and Site Layout

The roof garden is located on the south side of the hospital complex, three floors above the ground. On the north side, it is bounded by a four-story wing containing patient rooms and offices in the maternity department. On the other three sides, the garden looks out onto expansive views: to the east, the wooded and partly residential Berkeley Hills; to the south,

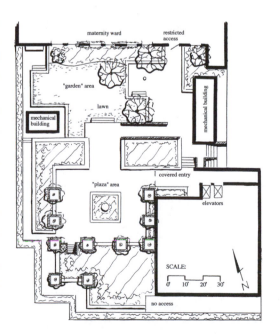

Map 7–1:
*The Roof Garden, Illustrative Plan*

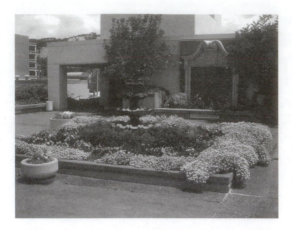

Berkeley residential neighborhoods of single-family houses; to the west, a panoramic view of San Francisco Bay, the city of San Francisco, the Golden Gate Bridge, and the hills of Marin County.

The garden consists of several distinct sub-areas. Upon emerging from the elevator, one walks out onto a square, brick-paved plaza bounded by flowered planters with seat-height concrete edges, and eight small carob trees in concrete boxes. In the middle of the plaza is a square flower bed with a small fountain at its center (see Photo 7–1). On a wall bounding the eastern edge of this plaza, two ornate columns and a crest that formed the entrance to the hospital in 1928 were saved and placed here after the building was demolished in 1983. The feeling of this sub-area is of an urban plaza, with users sitting around the edge, exposed to each other.

The second major section of the roof garden is four steps below the plaza and has more of a garden feel to it (see Photo 7–3). A small brick- and concrete-paved plaza accessed from a door in the maternity wing is bounded by seat-height concrete planters and a large raised lawn. Three maple trees offer some shade on hot days, and a lush expanse of red and purple climbing bougainvillaea has grown to the third floor of the adjacent building (see Photo 7–5).

A third, small and hidden section of the garden consists of a walkway behind the planters on the west and south sides of the roof. Movable garden chairs have been carried here for a very private sitting, viewing, and conversation setting (see Photo 7–4).

A fourth sub-area is under a building overhang by the elevators where a drink and a snack machine are located. As discussed in a later section, this small "anteroom" to the garden proper is well used because it is near the elevators and near snack machines; on hot days it is sheltered from the sun's glare; on frequent windy days it is screened from the breeze.

## Ambience and Microclimate

The background hum of a large air-conditioning/heating unit is ever-present as one enters the garden, though it is not unduly intrusive everywhere, depending on where one sits. One is aware of bird-song, and in the large plaza area, of the sounds of the fountain. On a breezy day, the rustle of trees and vines is a soothing backdrop for garden-users. The garden is high enough off the ground so that traffic cannot be heard. Apart from the sounds of an occasional plane or helicopter, the roof garden is very quiet and peaceful. When seated in most parts of the garden, the views over the city are screened by planting, and one has the sense of being in a secluded city garden.

A design factor that may inhibit use is the lack of elements to ameliorate the wind or bright sun. For perhaps half of the year, it is warm enough to sit outside, and, depending on the time of day, many would prefer to sit in the shade. The choice of planting in the main plaza — short, squat carob trees — was a poor one; they create very little shade. The roof tends to

Map 7–2:
*The Roof Garden, Experiential Analysis*

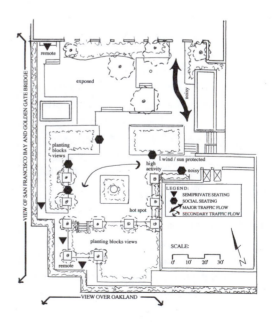

be more windy than the adjacent streets. A screened area offering shelter from the prevailing winds would have been a welcome addition.

## Garden Use

Compared to two other sites discussed in case studies in this report (Kaiser Walnut Creek and the Comfort Garden at San Francisco General Hospital), the roof garden at Alta Bates is relatively under-used. In eight hours of observation at the Kaiser site, there were 251 user-observations recorded; at San Francisco General, the number was 596. The number at Alta Bates was 154. This relative lack of use can be explained by a number of factors: A roof garden is a "terminus" location — most users go there to be there, they don't pass through it on the way to somewhere else; a roof garden tends to be more exposed to the elements than a garden at grade; the garden at Alta Bates is not publicized and is out of the way.

**TABLE 7–1**

*Percentage of User-Observations Recorded for Each Activity*

|  | Percent |
|---|---|
| Talk with colleagues or friends | 34 |
| Eat and/or drink | 24 |
| Smoke | 21 |
| Read, write | 8 |
| Look at the view | 6 |
| Sleep, doze, sunbathe | 5 |
| Work | 2 |

(Total number of user-observations: 154)

The most frequent pattern of use was for a person to walk from the elevator and find a place to sit while smoking a cigarette, or to enjoy a soft drink purchased from a machine near the elevator, or to eat a brown-bag lunch. Since the cafeteria is three floors down and almost a block away, it was very rare to see people arrive with their meal on a tray. Those arriving for a short break tended to cluster around the vending machines beneath a building overhang; it was here that most socializing took place. Those coming to the garden for a longer period tended to sit alone on the concrete seating bounding the main, brick-paved

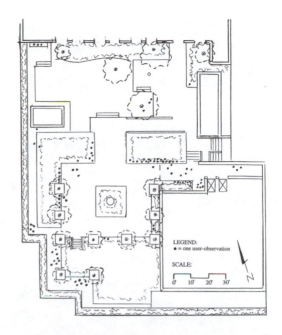

Map 7–3:
*The Roof Garden, Stationary Users*

plaza or to walk very purposefully to what appears to be a favorite seat or bench in more remote and hidden corners of the garden. The latter clearly came to be alone and often dozed, sunbathed, looked at the view, or meditated. Sixty percent came to the garden alone; 21 percent came in pairs, usually to eat lunch together. The 18 percent observed in groups were those who met each other while taking a break or stopped to chat for a while.

One of the disadvantages of the garden design for people in groups of two or more, or for those who want to *choose* where they sit, is the lack of movable seating. There were only five movable white plastic garden chairs (and three movable round tables), whereas there was more than 300 linear feet of concrete planter-edge seating. Not only were the chairs with backs more comfortable, but also they could be moved into the shade or sun, depending on the weather; they could be moved to sit and look at the view, or to join a friend at a table (see Photo 7–2). Considering the very secure location of the roof garden and the unlikelihood of anything being stolen, it is surprising that more movable seating has not been provided.

Those who were observed walking through the garden (one-fourth of the total) tended to move on one route — from the maternity wing exit to the vending machines, or from the elevator to the maternity wing — and not to spend any time in the garden.

Photo 7–2:
*Movable chairs
allow this staff
person to create a
private setting for
a lunch break.*

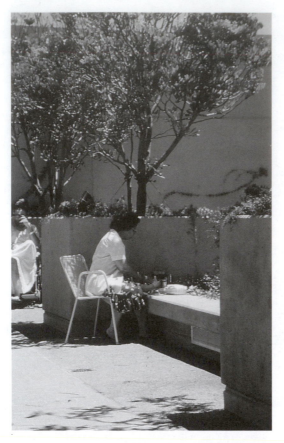

ing, talking, eating, strolling, and "outdoor therapy." Most came alone and stayed alone during their break; some joined colleagues whom they encountered in the garden. There is no lack of places to sit, though there is a lack of movable chairs, which people liked to take to a preferred location — into the shade, into the sun, to a more secluded setting.

## What Happens to People on the Roof Garden

When asked, "Do you feel any different after you've spent time in the garden?" all but one of the 36 interviewed reported a positive change in mood (see Table 7–2).

### Table 7–2

*Percent of Respondents Reporting Various Types of Mood Change*

|  | Percent |
|---|---|
| Calmer, more contented, more relaxed, less stressed | 80 |
| Refreshed, stronger | 33 |
| Better, more positive | 22 |
| Escape from work | 22 |
| Moves me, a religious connection | 8 |
| Helps me think through problem | 5 |
| Time passes more quickly | 3 |
| No difference in mood | 3 |

(Number of respondents: 36)

## Interviews with Users of the Roof Garden

Thirty-six people who were spending time in the garden were interviewed, half men and half women. Of these, 29 were staff, 3 were visitors, 2 were outpatients and 2 inpatients. It was disappointing to see so few in- and outpatients using this attractive facility. This is due in part to lack of information about its existence and in part to security measures following the kidnapping of a newborn baby several years ago. The main door onto the garden is now inaccessible to all but maternity patients and their visitors.

The garden was used predominantly by staff. A third of those we interviewed reported using the garden several times each day, and one-fourth came once a day. The primary use of the garden was either for a quick break with coffee, soft drink, or cigarette (almost one-half used the garden at some time for this less-than-10-minute break); or for a lunchtime or longer visit of 10–30 minutes.

When asked what they did in the garden, the most frequently cited activities were relax-

Many respondents referred to the pleasing *contrast* between the garden — open, sunny, colorful, "natural" — and the environment inside the hospital. For example, a man whose wife had just given birth had come to the garden three times that day: "I feel more relaxed. It's mostly because there aren't too many people out here. I'm a solitude kind of person. The sunlight is nice. The waiting room with fluorescent light sucks the energy out of you." Many felt the garden helped them calm down or relax from stressful situations at work. A female employee who uses the garden every day responded: "It's a place for meditation and relaxation. It's real tranquil. Because I work in the radiation department in the basement, I feel like one of the Mole People; I come out for sun. It's a big mental, emotional lift."

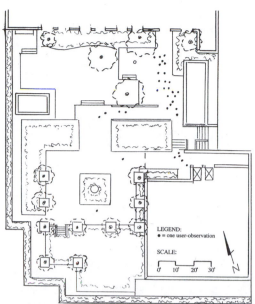

LEGEND:
● = one user-observation

SCALE:
0'  10'  20'  30'

Map 7–4:
*The Roof Garden,
Users Passing
Through*

For many people, the garden provides a welcome relief from the stress of constant interaction with people. A female employee who visits the garden two or three times a week remarked: "I'm at peace — you can see the birds and the water. I feel a sense of meditation; I feel better. Breathing the fresh air helps clear my head even if I need to scream or run in place. It's getting away from people, from work. The air itself helps me revive."

Many employees thought of the garden as "an escape." A male employee who uses the garden every day said: "It's an excellent area for relaxation even if it's only for a short time. Five minutes out here is better than an hour in the cafeteria. Its calming influence creates a sense of separation from the hospital that a recreation room wouldn't provide. It's a complete getaway."

Though relatively few patients used the garden, responses from two who did are indicative of what such a space can mean to someone who is sick or in recovery. A female inpatient responded: "I feel more normal here. I felt really depressed in there; I was getting real teary. You go from having control of your life to less control. Out here you're on your own; there's time to forget about it. You feel relieved from all the medical aspects of your case. You come out here and it's more holistic, more natural."

A female outpatient was waiting for an appointment and recalled practicing walking on the lawn as an inpatient recovering from an accident: "When you're in the hospital it's easy to get caught up in that whole sick vibe. When you come out here it's life, a surrender — that you're still breathing, you're still alive."

For all but one of the 36 people interviewed, the garden helped evoke a positive change in mood. Staff members returned to work feeling more relaxed; in- and outpatients felt calmer outside the normal hospital environment.

## What Specific Characteristics of the Garden Helped Bring About a Mood Change

Most people were quite forthright about what — in particular — in the garden helped them feel better. Overall, aspects of planting (flowers, "greenery," colors, seasonal changes) were by far the most often cited (see Table 7–3). Indeed, it is the flowers, lawn, trees, shrubs that make this a garden and not just a rooftop space. The fountain, though small, is centrally placed and audible from seating places in the main plaza section. Importantly, it also offers water to birds, which frequently come to drink and bathe. Some have made nests and raised their young in the roof garden.

**TABLE 7–3**

*Percent of Respondents Who Name These Qualities as Helpful in Attaining a Mood Change*

| | Percent |
|---|---|
| Flowers, colors | 67 |
| Openness, views | 36 |
| Greenery, seasonal change, "nature" | 33 |
| Water, fountain | 31 |
| Peacefulness, no traffic noise | 31 |
| Escape, privacy, secret places | 28 |
| Sun, light, fresh air | 28 |
| Birds | 25 |
| Design features (textures, shapes) | 19 |
| Sounds, smells | 14 |
| Management policy (smoking okay) | 8 |
| Places to sit, companionship | 5 |
| Don't know | 3 |
| No answer | 3 |

(Number of respondents: 36)

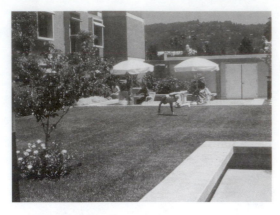

Photo 7–3:
*The "garden" area provides an expanse of lawn for more casual use, and children's play.*

Features that are specifically characteristic of a roof garden were also important — views, openness, fresh air, breezes, and being away from traffic noise.

A female employee who uses the roof garden several times a day responded enthusiastically:

> It's a whole different environment. The birds, the flowers, the sunshine, the fresh air, being away from the work environment. It helps build relationships. Everyone who comes up, we've gotten to know each other. It's a place to meet people. I feel very fortunate to have this. Sometimes, in the evening, the sun is setting. It's a wonderful experience. I have a lot of pride in this garden. I tell patients about it, and new employees when I'm orienting them.

An outpatient who was in the garden for the second time in one day also appreciated the birds, the fresh air, the greenery, the wind blowing, but especially the colorful flowers: "I do energy work with colors and chakras. Different colors arouse different emotions. You have all the colors of the chakras out here. It soothes you down. ... I can come out here and be still." A woman employee said that some of the flowers took her back to her childhood and their colors made her think about dress material for her granddaughters.

A female employee who comes to the garden to relax, stroll, eat, and "center myself" was especially articulate about which characteristics helped change her mood.

> The most important thing for me is the fountain because I love the sound of water and it attracts birds. Then, there's the greenery and flowers. And a third component — the design is pleasing to the eye: There's a combination of shapes and sizes; the brick gives a warm feel. ... I like the

nooks and crannies so you can have a place to be alone. As an employee in healthcare, you're constantly giving, interacting. It's important to have a place to recharge.

## TABLE 7–4

*Percent of Respondents Who Named These Impediments to Using the Garden*

|  | Percent |
|---|---|
| Work schedule | 44 |
| Weather | 33 |
| No impediments | 28 |
| Distance, difficult access | 8 |
| Didn't know it was here | 5 |

(Number of respondents: 36)

It was primarily work schedules and the weather that inhibited people from coming to the garden as much as they would like. We suspect, however, that many nonusers do not come to the garden because they don't know of its existence.

## TABLE 7–5:

*Percent of Respondents Who Desired These Changes*

|  |  | Percent |
|---|---|---|
| Practical changes |  | 52 |
| More movable chairs | 25 |  |
| More tables | 8 |  |
| Food cart | 5 |  |
| Drinking fountain | 5 |  |
| Shelter | 5 |  |
| Outdoor pager | 3 |  |
| Change nothing |  | 50 |
| Planting changes |  | 11 |
| Aesthetic improvements |  | 8 |
| Better maintenance and access |  | 8 |

(Number of respondents: 36)

When asked if there was anything they would like to see changed on the roof garden, one-half said, "Nothing!" But a similar proportion voiced a variety of pragmatic changes that would make the space more usable. Principal among those was the desire for more movable tables and chairs, particularly the latter. This was very apparent as we observed people searching for a chair so they could join others at a table or sit with their feet up on one of the planting edges. With only five movable chairs, they were in great demand. Observations made by William Whyte in his film on the use of Manhattan plazas (*The Social Use of Small Urban Spaces*) suggest that people just like to be able to *move* a chair in a public space, even if only a foot or two, perhaps to have a sense of control over their environment. Apart from these movable chairs, all the seating on the roof garden comprised concrete edges to planters without backs.

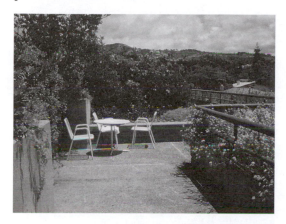

The fact that people often clustered around the vending machines under a concrete building overhang was in part due to lack of shade in the garden and — on windy days — lack of shelter. Several people requested shelter and more shade trees. A drinking fountain, a food cart, and an outdoor pager (for medical staff on call) were other practical suggestions. For the most part, however, users were well pleased with the garden. Aesthetic improvements were voiced by relatively few, but were worded quite vehemently.

A man visiting his wife in the hospital wanted "a pond with koi or goldfish where you can watch something methodical, take your mind off things." A young male outpatient visiting the garden for the first time had a lot to say:

> I would have made the area around the fountain round — there are a lot of rough edges. It would be nice to have an herbal section since we're in Berkeley, maybe a fragrance section. It would also be nice to have some unusual trees. It looks like someone went to the nursery and said, 'I'll have six of those.' It needs a canopied section for shade ... and some healing sculptures — man-

dalas, Buddha, Gaia — something relevant to healing.

## Conclusion

There is no doubt that for those who use it, the roof garden at Alta Bates facilitates relaxation and reduces stress. It was particularly beneficial to hospital employees, who reported returning to their work refreshed and more centered. A male employee who uses the garden every day as a "getaway for stress relief" reported: "You can come out here and meditate whether it's work related or stuff I'm dealing with at home. I can come out here and think about things and then go back in and be more productive." A female employee who occasionally visits the garden to eat lunch or talk with colleagues felt strongly that "all workplaces should have something like this — a place to go outside where it's quiet and pleasing to the eye, and sheltered. I think gardens are beneficial. I don't think fluorescent light and artificial air are healthy. If you go out and get away from that environment, you're more productive."

The fact that many of our respondents used the words "more productive," or implied such an outcome, is an indication that such outdoor spaces are not merely "cosmetic extras" but should be intrinsic components of every working environment. The health of the staff is as important as that of the patients. One male doctor who worked part time at another hospital remarked that at the other facility, there were plants but no places to sit. "Here I sit and smoke one cigarette and I don't need another to relax me." While smoking is not beneficial to health, if the garden enables an employee to

Photo 7–4:
*A private spot with a view is often sought out by staff.*

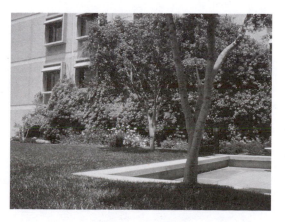

Photo 7–5:
*Magenta and orange bougainvillaea climbing the wall provides a very colorful backdrop for the garden, and is an attractive feature for the patients confined to their beds in the adjacent rooms.*

relax with one cigarette rather than two, that is certainly a benefit.

While staff were certain of its benefits to themselves, they also felt strongly about the value of a garden for patients. A female employee who thought of the garden as a "natural haven in an unnatural setting" remarked at the end of her interview: "I've worked in long-term-care settings for the past eight years. Of all the places that need cost-effective gardens, those are crying out for something like this — for patients and staff. With the aging of America and increased use of convalescent facilities, it is important for those places to have gardens."

A male employee used to bring patients out for certain therapies, but now time doesn't allow it. He felt the garden was an important setting for people who are dying: "We've brought patients out here to die because the family asked for it. They were able to die in peace without the critical-care setting. When the family decides to 'let go,' we'll jump through hoops to let a patient come out here to die."

A female employee who uses the garden every day to relax, eat, meditate, and exercise summed it up by saying, "It's like time has stopped, like a vacuum, a quiet space. I'm really glad it's here, it gives me an 'out.' I close my eyes and listen to the water as if I'm hearing a stream or a brook. ... I can get away from the downstairs hustle and bustle. It's the best thing about Alta Bates."

Or, as a male employee who was too busy to be interviewed remarked as he made his way to the elevator, "I'll tell you this ... if it weren't for the garden, we'd all be on Prozac."

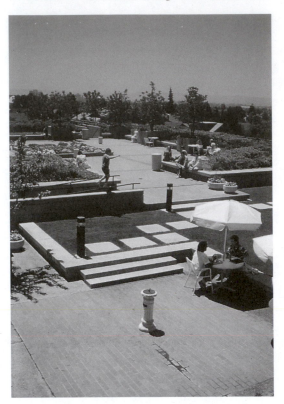

Photo 7–6:
*The absence of shade and wind protection is apparent in this overview of the roof garden.*

# 8. CASE STUDY: KAISER PERMANENTE MEDICAL CENTER, WALNUT CREEK, CALIFORNIA:
## *Central Garden*

## Physical Elements and Site Layout

The central garden at Kaiser, Walnut Creek, is the largest of the landscapes in this study. Designed around two heritage valley oaks, the garden is spacious enough to accommodate in addition several mature sycamores, pines, box elders, sweet gums, and olive trees. Under the tree canopies are undulating borders of shrubbery and large expanses of lawn punctuated with movable picnic tables as well as fixed benches.

The garden is crisscrossed with paths, being anchored at one corner by the main hospital entrance while the multistory parking structure is situated diagonally opposite. The hospital extends its single-story arms out to encompass the east and south sides of the space with sliding glass doors and windows that lead directly into patient rooms. These wings house post-op patients and some pediatric and orthopedic patients. The length of stay is sometimes as long as three weeks; however, the average stay was reported to be three days. One of the wings is being shut down for renovations and was at 50 percent occupancy at the time of the study. These patients' rooms are buffered from the larger lawn areas by a wide, covered arcade, low shrubs, and semiprivate seating areas.

The other two sides of the garden are filled in with a four-story outpatient medical building to the north, and the two-story cafeteria building and single-story outpatient EKG center to the west. Due to the layout of the perimeter

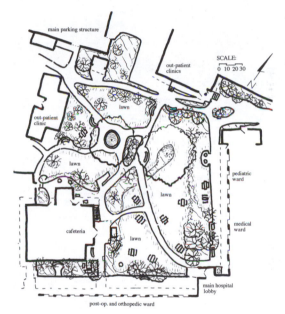

Map 8–1: *The Central Garden, Illustrative Plan*

buildings, people traverse the space almost continually, even in the rain and the near 100-degree temperatures common here, near California's Central Valley.

## Atmosphere and Ambience

Predictably idyllic weather through most of the year, though tending toward hotter temperatures, makes this open and airy garden space an inviting place. The evergreen plantings at eye level and below serve to provide a psychological screen from the low buildings. The trees comb the open sky, blowing in the breeze and providing homes for the birds that are always chirping. Squirrels scamper across the grass and chatter at passers-by from overhead limbs. The spreading

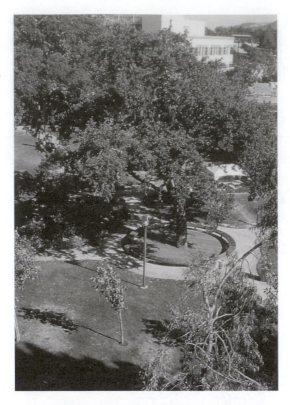

vation, 745 either stopped to talk, or sat eating, waiting, smoking a cigarette, or purposefully passing the time by strolling the grounds or playing.

The high number and diversity of the services surrounding the garden made it difficult to differentiate among visitors, outpatients, and nonmedical staff. However, we recorded that 29 percent of the users were medical staff, uniformed employees, or construction workers. Less than 2 percent were inpatients and the remaining 69 percent appeared to be visitors, outpatients, or nonmedical employees.

The proximity of the cafeteria contributed to the high number of people recorded eating or drinking (33 percent of the stationary users), in the same way that the overall hospital site planning dictated the large number of people moving through it.

## Interviews with Users of the Garden

A total of 50 people were interviewed in the garden; two-thirds of them were women. Of those interviewed, 27 were staff, 11 were visitors, 8 were outpatients, and 4 were inpatients. Almost half reported using the garden every day or several times a day; a third used it "occasionally." With the presence of picnic tables, ample seating (see Map 8–2), and an adjacent cafeteria, it is not surprising to find that one-fifth reported spending periods of more than

oaks lend their grand dignity to the space, providing a beautiful focal point from afar and the comfort of protected seating beneath. Visitors were observed bringing their dogs to visit with inpatients on the lawn, and the feeling is truly one of an enjoyable suburban park.

Many seating options are provided, with benches located along the walkways, some in the sun and others in dappled shade. There are permanent stone tables and stool-like seats in clusters, and wooden picnic tables that change orientation with the lawn-mowing schedule. There is a well-used covered patio with tables and chairs directly outside of the cafeteria's plate glass windows. There are two maps for newcomers, and a pay phone. Ashtrays and trash cans abound, and the grounds have a clean and tidy appearance.

Map 8–2:
*The Central Garden, Experiential Analysis*

## Garden Use

Movement through the garden was constant and of such an intense rate (see Map 8–3) that the speed of the observer in tracking and recording this activity became a limiting factor during the first phase of the study. The passers-by are underrepresented perhaps by 15 percent. However, of the 1251 people recorded during the two mornings and two afternoons of obser-

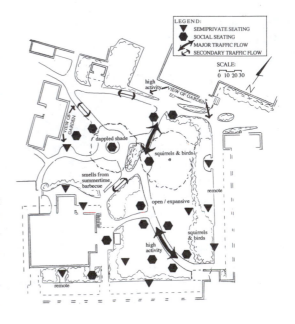

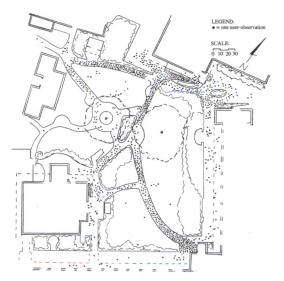

Map 8–3:
*The Central
Garden,
Users Passing
Through*

30 minutes in the garden, and nearly three-fourths took breaks of 10 to 30 minutes. This contrasts with Alta Bates' roof garden, in which relatively few used the garden for 5- to 10-minute breaks.

### TABLE 8–1

*Percent of Respondents Using Gardens for Various Activities*

|  | Percent |
|---|---|
| Relaxing | 88 |
| Walking through | 84 |
| Eating | 82 |
| Talking | 70 |
| Strolling | 54 |
| Waiting | 52 |
| Outdoor therapy | 46 |
| Visiting with a patient | 42 |
| Kids playing | 18 |
| Attending a meeting | 16 |

(Number of respondents: 50)

While "relaxing" appeared high on the list here and at all the case study gardens, at this Kaiser facility a higher proportion than elsewhere reported using the garden for eating, visiting with a patient, watching their kids play, and attending an outdoor meeting. Almost half reported there were no impediments to their using the garden, and most of the remainder — as at other sites — reported weather and work as the only serious impediments.

The garden was highly regarded and appre-ciated by everyone we spoke with, especially by staff, who were thankful for the contrast between the indoor and outdoor environments. A female employee who comes out once or twice a day to relax, talk, eat, stroll or visit with a patient responded, "You can get away from the fluorescent lights, sounds, and smells of a hospital; listen to the birds, the breeze. It's a tremendous place to unwind."

### TABLE 8–2

*Percent of Respondents Who Named These Qualities as What They Liked Best*

|  | Percent |
|---|---|
| Trees, plants, flowers | 82 |
| Aesthetic attractiveness and design | 72 |
| Serenity, quiet, "escape" | 54 |
| Birds, squirrels, open air, sun | 50 |
| Expansiveness, open space | 8 |
| Human companionship | 4 |

(Number of respondents: 50)

Another employee uses the garden several times a day and loves the trees, plants, and animals: "I feed the squirrels and birds. I have two blue jays who come down to eat peanuts — and there's George the squirrel (I speak fluent squirrel!). I can recognize the baby squirrels even though they're now grown. I've even come here on my day off!"

Several people felt it looked like a park or "a country club." Employees especially appreciated its tranquillity:

I like the openness, the grass, birds, the breeze. Although there's a lot of people around, there's a quietness about it. It reminds me of a campus.

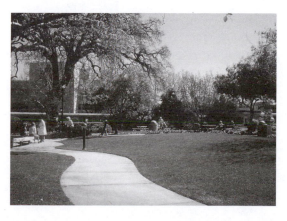

Photo 8–2:
*This walking route from the parking structure to the main hospital lobby is highly used. The multistory building is dwarfed by the tree and recedes, while the lawns create a soothing green milieu.*

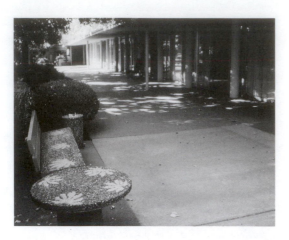

I like it when I do swing shift; at dusk you could imagine this is your backyard. I like the tranquillity. It has a certain peace about it.

Visitors and outpatients appreciated having a relaxing place in which to wait, and a female inpatient remarked:

I really hate hospitals a lot. I get tired of my room. It's so much nicer out here — I like seeing the grass and hearing the birds. I come out several times a day to sit or stroll or have a smoke. My favorite time is the evening when everything is really quiet. ... It's much better than sitting inside and watching the boob tube.

### TABLE 8–3

***Percent of Respondents Reporting Various Types of Mood Changes***

|  | Percent |
| --- | --- |
| Calmer, more relaxed | 86 |
| Stronger, refreshed | 24 |
| Escape from work | 18 |
| Moves me, a religious connection | 6 |
| Better, positive | 6 |
| No difference in mood | 6 |
| Helps me think through problems | 4 |

(Number of respondents: 50)

When we asked if people felt any different after spending time in the garden, the most frequent and consistent response was: "Yes — more relaxed." A garden and a hospital are almost polar opposites on a continuum from controlled to natural, from stressful to relaxing. It is small wonder that staff and employees felt so passionately about this garden in the midst of their work environment:

I work in the operating room. We have no windows; it's very cold with artificial light. This is the complete opposite — it gives me a lift to come out in the natural light.

I feel more calm, more relaxed. If you want to get away from things, just sit under a tree and reflect — things usually get better.

It's very soothing because it's so different from the interior of the building, which is stressful. This is a complete opposite.

I'm back to being me again. This is absolutely my little spot to get centered and heal myself.

I work in ICU, which is like a hellhole. For the first four hours I just run. Sitting out in the warm sun is like therapy to me. I can relax, gather my thoughts. I feel like I have my head screwed on straight.

Visitors and patients who used the garden felt strongly about how this place facilitated a change in mood. An outpatient who told us she brought visitors from Europe to show them what a nice hospital looks like remarked:

It doesn't feel, smell, or look like a hospital. Coming to a hospital scares and worries people. Being in the garden before or after visiting the doctor is good, regardless of what you find out. I feel more relaxed.

A woman waiting in the garden while her husband was at an appointment responded, "I feel more peaceful out here. I get very tired waiting for them to tell me how he's doing. I'm not as tired outdoors."

A woman in labor was strolling through the garden, waiting for the birth of her child. "This is my first time here. I've been admiring the trees, the landscape, the quietness, the birds. It's really relaxing — when I'm not having a contraction."

A male inpatient was occupying one of the rooms that open out onto the garden:

I really hate hospitals, but having this room — it doesn't bother me so much. I feel a little easier, a little more relaxed outdoors. When people come to see me, we can sit out here and it makes a much nicer visit. It's really relaxing to know that other people enjoy it, too.

People had no trouble "connecting" their change in mood with specific characteristics of the garden, even if — as some said — they hadn't consciously thought about this before. For many, it was a whole range of elements. For a male employee who used the garden at least once a day it was "the shade from the trees, the breeze, the birds, the colors, the sounds of the leaves, the squirrels running up and down the trees, no litter in sight."

**TABLE 8–4**

*Percentage of Respondents Who Named These Qualities as Helpful in Attaining Mood Change*

| | | Percent |
|---|---|---|
| Trees and Plants | | 86 |
| Trees | 36 | |
| Greenery | 18 | |
| Nature | 14 | |
| Colors | 10 | |
| Flowers | 6 | |
| Seasons | 2 | |
| Features involving auditory, olfactory, or tactile sensations | | 60 |
| Birds, squirrels | 24 | |
| Fresh air | 12 | |
| Shade | 10 | |
| Light and sun | 8 | |
| Sounds, smells | 6 | |
| Psychological/social aspects | | 64 |
| Peaceful | 18 | |
| Openness, largeness | 14 | |
| Escape | 10 | |
| Oasis | 8 | |
| Privacy | 6 | |
| Watching others, companions | 6 | |
| No traffic noise | 2 | |
| Visual qualities relating to more than plant materials | | 26 |
| Visually attractive design | 14 | |
| Variety | 10 | |
| Texture | 2 | |
| Practical features | | 26 |
| Places to sit | 12 | |
| Good maintenance | 6 | |
| Accessible | 4 | |
| Pathways and amenities | 4 | |
| Don't know; no answer | | 10 |

(Number of respondents: 50)

A female inpatient interviewed near her room particularly liked "listening to the birds; it's quiet here. I like to see other people sitting and relaxing on the benches. I can't get out there, but it's neat; it's really relaxing."

A visitor to the hospital who occasionally uses the garden liked "the landscaping, the birds. You can get a cup of coffee, sit back, and look at the trees. Every time I come, it's a different season. It takes your mind off whatever you're here for."

The huge oak trees elicited a lot of positive comment, particularly their size, their great age, the wildlife they harbored, and, for some, the memories they evoked. A male security guard who patrols the garden liked the tranquillity and peace "... and the large trees, when the wind blows through the branches. It's a sound I got used to as a kid growing up in the Arizona countryside."

For others it was the oasislike quality of the space that helped evoke a change in mood. A male employee who comes out to sit and eat several times a day feels calmer as a result and attributes that to "the trees, the grass, birds, animals — its like an oasis among the concrete, yet it's close to whatever you need. You have to stay conscious because you can get into a mood and forget about the time."

A male outpatient also liked the enclosed feeling: "I liked the fact that it's surrounded by buildings ... it's kind of nestled, protected. But it's not too close to the buildings; you don't feel you're in an urban park."

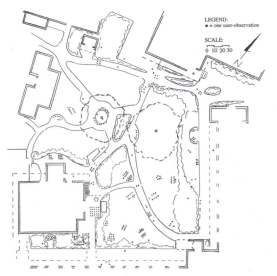

LEGEND:
● = one user-observation

SCALE:
0 10 20 30

Map 8–4:
*The Central Garden, Stationary Users*

Though this space is not large by park standards, we got the sense that people *experienced* it as spacious because of the planting that screened some of the surrounding buildings; because — by hospital standards — it *is* a large open space; and because for some, it is such a contrast to the small spaces in which they live and work.

A female employee confided:

> When I work evenings, I come here two hours early and just *sit* here! In my life, this is a vast space. I live in a little condo, work in a little office in surgery. This is like a vast open space to me! The patients come out here all the time — pregnant women waddle around. They say, "This is such a great space, so soothing. Who'd believe this was here?"

Finally, for a few people, it is not so much the trees, the fresh air, animals, and openness that help change their mood, but the companionship and good spirits of other people in the garden, particularly, it seems, the gardeners. One employee who admitted, "I'd be out here all day long if I could," added, "The gardeners keep us laughing all the time. They do such a good job, keeping the garden. It's a joy to have them out there." In creating a garden for therapeutic outcomes it would pay not only to design it with care, but also to select maintenance staff for their sensitivity and good humor.

Just under half wanted no changes made to the garden. Others wanted to see planting improvements — especially more flowers, the addition of a water feature, a drinking fountain, more tables and seating. Compared with the other sites we observed, Kaiser has provided well for smokers. A small three-sided, roofed structure with comfortable chairs inside was erected in

spring 1995 for the convenience of smokers who need to come outside. While this looks onto the garden, the smokers don't annoy nonsmokers by sitting next to them on a garden bench.

### TABLE 8–5

***Percent of Respondents Who Desired These Changes***

| | | Percent |
|---|---|---|
| Change nothing | | 46 |
| Planting changes | | 22 |
|    More flowers, color | 16 | |
|    More trees, shade | 6 | |
| Aesthetic and planning improvements | | 16 |
|    Add a water feature | 8 | |
|    Make it larger | 4 | |
|    Create a Japanese garden | 2 | |
|    Move freeway | 2 | |
| Practical changes | | 14 |
|    Drinking fountain | 4 | |
|    More tables | 2 | |
|    More seating | 2 | |
|    A shelter for rainy weather | 2 | |
|    More designated smoking | 2 | |
|    Add sports facilities | 2 | |
| Policy changes | | 12 |
|    Better maintenance | 6 | |
|    Ban smoking | 2 | |
|    Stop removing trees | 2 | |
|    Less construction | 2 | |

(Number of respondents: 50)

## Conclusion

Hospitals are obviously associated in most people's minds with illness, accidents, and death. It is clear from observing — and talking with — people in the garden at Kaiser Walnut Creek that the presence of *life* just outside is enormously therapeutic. The trees, the birds, the squirrels, children playing — all remind people that "life goes on." An outpatient waiting for her appointment felt "rested spiritually" in the garden: "It's a privilege to be here. Look at this incredible oak tree — it's a universe in itself." Several patients and employees mentioned the fact that the garden made *this* Kaiser facility unique and that they used (or had taken a job at) Walnut Creek specifically

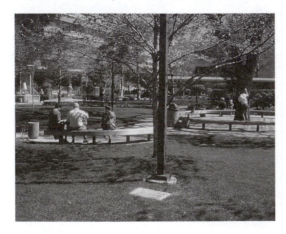

Photo 8–4:
*Casual seating along the walkway provides a convenient resting spot. Wood decking and a circular bench protect the roots of one heritage oak while providing seating with an array of vistas and informal play space for children.*

because of its soothing milieu. One of the gardeners told us, "They call this Kaiser 'the country club.'"

One employee who had worked in many medical facilities since 1959 rated this — because of the garden — as one of the best. And a male employee who uses the garden every day, sometimes to do work-related reading, summed it up with:

> I work in the operating room — no windows. The diurnal cycle is interrupted. Out here, it's open to the sky. It fits with the holistic idea of what I think healthcare is. It's not only medicine and physical treatment; you also have that part that's unique to the individual called the soul. This garden helps to revive that.

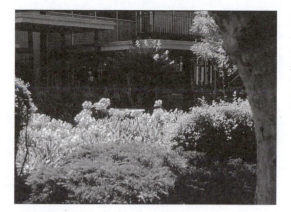

Photo 8–5:
*A covered patio off the cafeteria provides shade and shelter for an outdoor eating area within the garden.*

# 9. CASE STUDY: CALIFORNIA PACIFIC MEDICAL CENTER, GARDEN CAMPUS, SAN FRANCISCO[1]:
## *The Garden*

RESPONDING TO THE need to rehouse the many patients displaced by the 1906 earthquake, the Home for the Incurables was opened on this site in 1915. In 1938 the facility changed hands, was renamed the Garden Nursing Home, and began providing an array of rehabilitative services ranging from cardiac and respiratory therapy through physical therapy and vocational counseling. Today this small private hospital for patients of moderate means is in transition. It currently offers post-acute care and hospice services to AIDS and other chronically ill patients. The average length of stay at Garden Campus is around 30 days.

The garden is now an important feature of this facility, but it also played a prominent role in the history of this site. Several photo albums kept by the administration track the various changes and momentous events. The staff here are proud of the garden, and it is an integral part of the hospital's identity.

## Physical Elements and Site Layout

The original garden was a formally laid out herb garden with lawns, circular paths, and larger shrubbery and trees around the perimeter. The plan has been modified several times and now incorporates two glazed shelters with tables and chairs, two larger patio areas, one in the sun and one predominantly in the shade, and a volleyball/basketball court (see Photo

9–1). The garden has a mature feel, as much of the original perimeter planting has been retained. A large camphor tree dominates, along with other gnarled fruit trees and the vestiges of the formal yew and boxwood plantings. An addition to the west wing of the hospital added a long balcony off the day room on the third floor, which meets grade and leads down into the garden. In view of the balcony's location directly over the garden, and the direct pathway down to ground level, the balcony was included in our observations as part of the garden (see Photo 9–5). This sunny elevated spot proved to be the most used area, offering

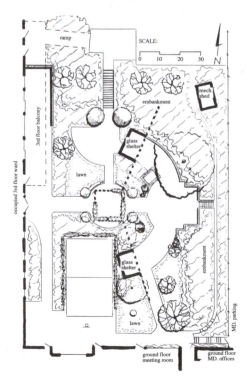

Map 9–1:
*The Garden, Illustrative Plan*

---

[1] Due to hospital remodeling during the research period, this case study is descriptive only.

Photo 9–1:
*This interesting
and eclectic garden
offers a variety of
uses from active to
passive. Particu-
larly interesting is
the incorporation
of a basketball/
volleyball court,
which is highly
used by the chil-
dren of patients
and visitors.*

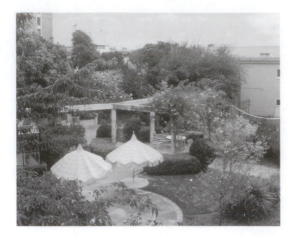

accessibility, wind protection, and a view of the entire garden.

There are four main access points in the garden: a gate to the physicians' parking lot, one door off each of the second-floor wings of the building (see Photo 9–2), and the path down from the balcony off the third-floor day room (see Photo 9–3). Due to current renovation, the hospital houses only 18 patients, all on the third floor of this west wing. Accessing the ground level of the garden from this ward necessitates either descending 17 concrete steps down the slope adjacent to the balcony, or using the main interior elevator and passing through the empty second floor to the garden doors. The garden is approximately 95 feet by 135 feet, with about one-third of the area being a heavily planted embankment.

## Atmosphere and Ambience

Located between a residential and retail/small commercial neighborhood, the 2½-story, L-shaped hospital building nestles into the southwestern slope of Laurel Heights in San Francisco. The garden is on the uphill side, behind the building; while breezes eddy through the space, the prevailing winds are thwarted by the hospital itself. The freshness of the salt sea air is a reminder of the proximity of the ocean, and even on sunny days the rhythmic sound of a nearby foghorn reminds one of the preciousness of this secluded and relatively protected spot.

This entire facility has an intimate feeling, with the street facade resembling an old expensive hotel rather than a medical center. The garden in turn creates a feeling of intima-

cy, being bounded by the building on two sides and steep slopes of mature planting on the north and eastern edges. The small number of patients and the temporarily empty floors, as well as the mix of design styles and utilitarian functions within the garden, contribute to the timeless and almost "forgotten" feeling of this space.

## Garden Use

Awareness of the garden and pride in it contribute to the continued utilization of this outdoor space, despite the serious accessibility issues. During the 12 hours of observation, 131 user-observations were recorded. In addition to the staff using the garden for their breaks, half of the reports were of patients and guests coming out for strolls and visits. On the weekend, the space was used by children playing while family members visited with others inside, and during one of the observation periods, the garden was being set up for a volunteer appreciation party later that afternoon.

The staff have commented upon the drop in the use of the garden since the reduction in the number of patients, and the subsequent closing of all but the third floor of one wing. However, during our observation the staff were seen to encourage patients to spend time outside, and they themselves would come to the balcony rail for a glance out and a deep breath before returning to their tasks inside. The feeling about the garden is demonstrated by an episode that took place while three employees were on a break. They became concerned about the health of the rosemary

Photo 9–2:
*Appealing and
convenient access
at ground level
draws people into
the garden. Wide,
smooth walkways
facilitate use by
patients on gurneys
or in wheelchairs.*

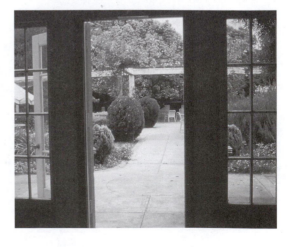

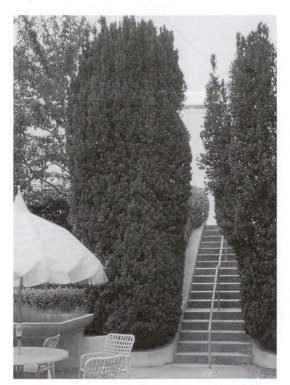

ground cover on the slope below the balcony on which they were standing. They took it upon themselves to slosh water out of a plastic bin, onto the plants below, making several trips in to the sink, to make sure that they got enough.

The layout of the hospital grounds is such that it is equally convenient to travel inside as outside when moving between most destinations. The significance of this is that the people observed passing through the garden were most likely doing this as a reflection of their preference for an outdoor route (see Map 9–2). Although most of the users of the garden were stationary, a fifth of the uses recorded in the garden were children playing. Although playing was recorded at all of the case study sites, this site presented not only the largest percentage of this activity, but also children playing for the longest time, and on their own. Their parent-visitors were observed to come to the balcony railing from time to time to check on their children, and then return to the bedside. The children, however, happy to be playing, entertained themselves for extended periods of time. The easy observation from the balcony (see Photo 9–1) and the secure nature of the garden both contributed to this phenomenon.

## Interviews with Users of The Garden

Seven people were interviewed while spending time in the garden at this site. Of these, five were women and two were men; four were staff and three were visitors. Only one patient used the garden during the interview periods despite the fact that almost a fifth of the users during the observation period were inpatients. This patient was unable to speak due to a recent stroke, but his wife did participate in the interviews. The medical staff reported that with the downsizing of the hospital and the relocation of the post-op patients, the general health of the patient population had declined during the study.

During the interview phase of the study, the majority of patients were confined to their beds and unable to be moved into the garden. Despite this situation, we were able to record the comments of several visitors and staff regarding patient use of the garden. One nurse supervisor told of patients requesting to be moved into the garden just before they die, so that they may spend their last minutes outside. Another reported that when the hospital was full, and there were more healthy AIDS patients, "there were always people in the garden: patients alone or with visitors, having barbecues and such."

Of the seven visitors and staff that were interviewed, all reported that it was a relaxing en-

Photo 9–3:
*Old yews, boxwood hedges, and formal stairways contribute to an atmosphere of timeless elegance.*

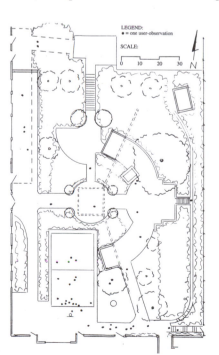

Map 9–2:
*The Garden, Users Passing Through or Playing*

Map 9–3:
*The Garden,
Stationary Users*

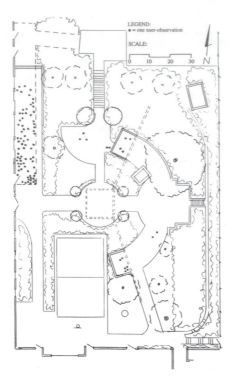

vironment. One staff member indicated that she was not able to relax in the garden because her focus was on the patients rather than on herself:

> It is quiet and peaceful ... (but) if you go out with the patient, you don't think of yourself, you are thinking of the patient.

## What Users Liked Best About The Garden

The most attractive aspects of the garden for the users were the quiet atmosphere and the sense of being removed from the hospital (see Photo 9–4). The plants and flowers were credited with providing this feeling. One employee commented:

> It's nice looking at the flowers, getting out of that claustrophobic place. It's like a safe haven.

And another:

> It is serene, tranquil. Up here (on the balcony) you can hear the wind going through the trees and I like the sound of that.

## Impediments to Use and Desired Changes in The Garden

Interviewees were asked if there was "anything that prevents or inhibits you from coming here as much as you would like." Most people

responded that there was not anything. However, one employee was quite vocal about being "too damn busy ... most of the time patients can't be taken out here, there isn't time. ... If I do take a patient out I can't relax ... I have a lot of patients who can't do anything for themselves."

The only other impediment was mentioned by an employee who commented that he "can't play basketball at night."

More flowers, specifically fragrant flowers, followed by concerns expressed regarding the upkeep of the garden were the two predominant requests in response to the question, "Is there anything you would like to see changed or added?"

One employee commented:

> I hope they keep it up; more flowering plants with a nice aroma. You're dealing with a lot of elderly patients ... I wish more of the patients could get out here. That's why I pick the flowers for the patients. The jasmine is nice, the smell if we can get it to waft into the rooms. When you put jasmine under their nose, they just light up.

Another:

> I'd like to see more flowers, (but) ... they'd have to hire someone to take care of it.

Outdoor lighting was not directly mentioned by the users who were interviewed; however, two of the respondents referred to drawbacks that could be solved by providing illumination at night. In addition to the comment about playing basketball at night quoted above, another staff member said:

> I used to work the PM shift, and I didn't see it that much. The flowers ... I've always been an outdoors person ... it is a nice treat (to see them).

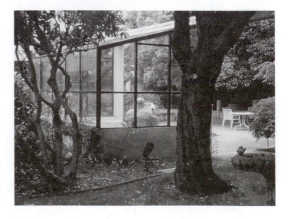

Photo 9–4:
*Glazed shelters
trap the heat, pro-
vide protection
from the breeze,
and create private
seating areas.
Features such as
this extend the use
of the garden into
many months of
the year.*

## What Happens to People in The Garden?

In response to the question "Do you feel any different after you've spent time in the garden?" all of the respondents said yes. Typical of comments from the staff was the nurse who said:

> (I feel) more relaxed, ready to go do my work. It gives me time to plan what I'm going to do when I get back to work; it clears my head."

and the doctor who said:

> If I play basketball, I feel very different, (and even) if I don't, and just go out for a few minutes, I feel better.

or the visitor who commented:

> Because his room is so small, it is relaxing to come out here, you catch air ... you don't know you are in a hospital.

## Specifically Helpful Characteristics

Several qualities of the garden were listed specifically in connection with the mood changes experienced by the users who were interviewed. Getting out into "fresh air and sunshine" and the trees and greenery were considered to be the major factors.

One staff member spoke of the greenery, and also of what the garden represents:

> The existence of plant life in general is a relaxant. And I think just that it (the garden) exists is heartwarming; someone cared enough to put it here.

A nurse spoke about her witnessing changes in the patients when she brings them out into the garden:

> To the patients, the garden is like a pet; it just makes them come up if they are depressed. You should see the expression on their faces, the body language. They just bloom up ... or it could make them sad, because it makes them think of their garden at home ... you have to watch their body language, how they breathe, their eyes. Greens do make a physical change.

## Conclusion

The nature of the Garden Campus, offering post-acute care and hospice services with a longer length of stay, directly influences the

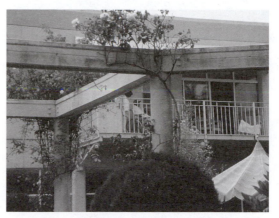

Photo 9–5:
*Patients on a sheltered balcony off the day room partake of the views and fragrances in the garden. The nursing staff often pop out to check on patients, while staying longer and enjoying the garden themselves on their breaks. Note the fragrant climbing rose on the arbor in the foreground.*

usage of the garden. The focus of the service provided here is necessarily more on "quality of life" than on the more immediate goal of medical stabilization at other institutions. Patients' emotions are addressed as a necessary part of the treatment agenda. Similarly, the significance of the ongoing support of visitors increases in proportion to the length of stay of the patients. The garden is a tremendous asset in allowing the residents and visitors to feel as comfortable as possible.

The reports of frequent family picnics in the garden, the intense use by children, the observations recorded by nurses of the emotional changes in the patients after spending time in the garden, all speak to the increased level of satisfaction and contentment that can be gained by having access to an outdoor space. Additionally, secondary benefits to the patient include the facilitation of more frequent and longer visits from family and loved ones, and being cared for by a staff who have the opportunity to rejuvenate themselves. In a demanding field such as healthcare, providing for the needs of all the participants, thereby maximizing all of the potential support-energy, is critically important.

The garden design and issues of accessibility play a significant role in the success of this garden space. The direct benefit of the garden for inpatients is tremendously increased by the availability of the outdoor balcony space immediately adjacent to the day room (see Map 9–3). Patients are brought out here to watch and enjoy the goings-on, while the proximity to the unit allows the staff to check on them regularly. When the second floor is again open, the accessibility off the

Map 9–4:
*The Garden,
Experiential
Analysis*

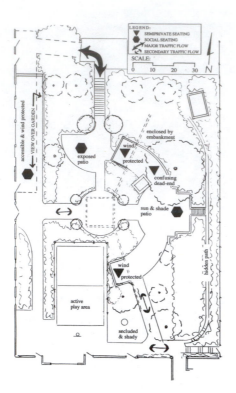

LEGEND:
SEMIPRIVATE SEATING
SOCIAL SEATING
MAJOR TRAFFIC FLOW
SECONDARY TRAFFIC FLOW
SCALE:
0    10    20    30    N

accessible & wind protected
VIEW OVER GARDEN

exposed
patio

wind/
protected

enclosed by
embankment

confusing
dead-end

sun & shade
patio

wind
protected

active
play area

hidden path

secluded
& shady

volleyball/basketball court is an additional draw for younger visitors, and is an outlet for the release of pent-up energy by the staff (see Map 9–4).

The garden at California Pacific's Garden Campus is a private and secluded oasis that has served many purposes over the years. Today it is again in transition, and like the institution itself is underutilized. Yet the sensitivity of the staff to the patients' enjoyment of the garden and its healing benefits, as well as the ethos and pride that this institution has in its namesake, continues to enable this facility to take the best advantage of this asset. (Is it a coincidence that of the units available, the one with the best access to the garden is the one remaining open?) The staff's patient loads have increased, and they feel overworked, yet they care for the garden on their breaks and come to work early to be able to enjoy it. Everyone encountered at this facility spoke of a desire to have the garden kept up as a contributing aspect of the hospital's treatment services. Indeed, plans are in the works to modify the garden to accommodate a future Alzheimer's unit.

*(At the time of printing, the Garden Campus site of California Pacific Medical Center has been temporarily closed in order to expedite the renovations and an anticipated merger.)*

west wing will offer the same advantage. Additionally, wind shelters, and patio surfaces and walls to reflect the heat are used by patients to moderate San Francisco's "natural air-conditioning." Thus, the patients have a way to stay warm without having to be directly exposed to the sun's rays. The unexpected existence of the

# 10. AGGREGATE DATA ANALYSIS OF THE CASE STUDY SITES

IN THE PREVIOUS chapters, four hospital garden case studies were presented. The use and therapeutic benefits of each of these exterior spaces was described. In this chapter the aggregate data is presented and analyzed to suggest overall trends. It is somewhat problematic to compile responses from differing sites, and there are a few qualifications that should be pointed out at this time.

While the differences in physical settings among the research sites add to the breadth of the study, they limit the aggregation of data. One aspect of this is the array of differing elements within the landscaped areas. This has been addressed in the analysis by focusing on categories of elements, rather than on specifics. For example, Kaiser Walnut Creek has two heritage oak trees that were mentioned by 36 percent of the people as a significant factor in their restorative process. There are relatively few blooming plants at Kaiser, and only 6 percent of the respondents mentioned the flowers. In contrast, San Francisco General has no heritage trees, however it had 35 different species of plants blooming at the time of the study. As might be expected, 42 percent of those people interviewed at San Francisco General mentioned the flowers, while only 4 percent mentioned the trees. For the purposes of the aggregate analysis, these two items have been grouped together under the heading of "trees and plants." A second difference among the four landscapes is the site layout. The garden's relationship to the buildings, how many access points there are, and the efficiency of travel through the space to interior destinations play a role in the way the garden is perceived and used. The focus of the aggregate analysis is therefore not on users moving through the space (though within the context of the individual site, this is significant).

## Aggregate Descriptive Data

One hundred and forty-three users were interviewed; 73 were female and 70 were male. 59 percent were employees, 26 percent were patients, and 15 percent were visitors. Nearly half of the respondents use the gardens every day, or several times a day.

**TABLE 10–1**

*Frequency of Garden Use*

|  | Percent |
| --- | --- |
| Several times per day | 30 |
| Occasionally/sometimes | 27 |
| Every day | 18 |
| 1-2 times per week | 14 |
| First time here | 11 |
| (Number of respondents: 143) | 100 |

We asked the users of the gardens to indicate one or more activities that they engaged in from a list of 10 options. All but 8 of the 143 users reported that they come to "relax." More than half of the users said that they come to talk, eat, stroll in the garden, and/or come for their own, undefined "outdoor therapy."

## TABLE 10–2

*Percent of Respondents Using Gardens for Various Activities*

| | Percent |
|---|---|
| Relax | 94 |
| Eat | 73 |
| Talk | 73 |
| Walk through | 68 |
| Stroll in the garden | 61 |
| Outdoor therapy | 53 |
| Wait | 38 |
| Visit with a patient | 36 |
| Let their children play here | 12 |
| Work-related meeting | 11 |

(Number of respondents: 143)

Ninety-five percent of the users of the garden reported that they "feel different" after spending time there. Just over three-quarters of the respondents described feeling more relaxed, and calmer. Somewhat less than a quarter of the users reported that they felt refreshed, rejuvenated, or stronger, while as many again spoke of being able to think more clearly, find answers, and felt more capable after being in the garden.

## TABLE 10–3

*Percent of Respondents Reporting Various Types of Mood Change*

| | Percent |
|---|---|
| More relaxed, less stressed, calmer, contented | 78 |
| Refreshed, rejuvenated, stronger | 25 |
| Able to think, find answers, cope | 22 |
| Pleased, better, more positive | 19 |
| Religious or spiritual connection | 6 |
| No difference in mood | 5 |

(Number of respondents: 143)

Of those specific characteristics or qualities of the garden named by users as helpful to them, two-thirds of the respondents mentioned trees, flowers, and plants. More than half mentioned features that involve either sounds or smells or tactile responses. Exactly half of those answering this question mentioned the psychological or social aspects of the space (it is peaceful; an escape from work; companionship; etc.).

# Comparative Analysis of the Aggregate Data

When looking at the activities in relation to the different types of users, there were some expected results and some associations that were not anticipated. Predictable responses were documented by those interviewees reporting that they came to the garden to "relax," to "stroll through," and to engage in "outdoor therapy." Each of these activities had a representative spread within the staff, patient, and visitor types. Also, as might be anticipated, differences in frequency of response arose for "work-related meetings," "eating," and "waiting." The staff reported the most instances of meeting and eating outdoors, with the visitors and patients tied at the top of the list of those who choose to wait in the garden.

Less expected were the results of inquiries regarding "talking" in the garden. The vast majority of employees reported that they talk while in the garden, as did close to two-thirds of the visitors. However, almost half of the patients said that they did *not* converse while they were there. One explanation for this may be that visitors specifically come to the hospital to talk and be with a patient, and staff are in a work environment where they have friends and acquaintances, whereas patients are isolated from their social milieu and know relatively few people. However, another possible explanation is that the situation of undergoing treatment at a medical facility may increase one's desire to get away and be alone.

The total number of interviewees who have used the hospital gardens as a play area for their children was relatively small. However, the rate of usage between the user types was nearly equal (see Figure 10–1). Similar results were recorded for those users who "visit with a patient." Again, the total percentage of users who visit with patients was not large, but the differences among rates of usage was revealing (see Figure 10–2). The fact that the employees engage in both of these activities indicates that the garden increases the number of options open to the staff. It gives employees more flexibility in their choices of how they work — whether they talk with patients indoors or outside — and also how they integrate their employment and their personal lives.

## TABLE 10–4

### Percent of Respondents Who Named These Qualities as Helpful In Attaining a Mood Change

| | Percent |
|---|---|
| Trees and plants | 69 |
| flowers, colors, greenery, heritage trees, being in nature, seasonal changes | |
| Features involving auditory, olfactory, or tactile sensations | 58 |
| birds/squirrels, wind/fresh air, water, quiet, light/sun, shade, fragrances | |
| Psychological or social aspects | 50 |
| peaceful, escape from work, openness/ large, privacy/secret places, oasis, companionship, watching others, knowing it is here | |
| Visual qualities relating to more than plant materials | 26 |
| attractive landscape design, views, variety of elements, textural contrast/ quality, differing shapes/sizes | |
| Practical features | 17 |
| seating, well maintained, accessibility, vending machines, smoking allowed, pathways | |
| No answer or "don't know" | 8 |

(Number of respondents: 143)

On one occasion a family was observed eating together in the garden. After playing with her two children for a period of time, the mother kissed them good-bye and said that she had to "go back to work now." Unusual though this may be, the interviews reveal that this is not an isolated incident. By using the garden in this way, the staff are taking the opportunity to satisfy their personal needs in a way that supports their work.

We also observed medical staff chatting with patients in the garden. Some of these appeared to be chance meetings. However, we did observe staff and patients coming out together and having what appeared to be a serious conversation. The opportunity for staff and patients to choose this outdoor setting for their meetings increases the degree of comfort

and often provides a level of privacy otherwise unavailable. This adds variation into the workday of the employee, and contributes to a sense of autonomy, so compromised for inpatients, as well.

When looking at the association between mood changes and user types, the results confirmed our expectations. Approximately equal proportions of visitors, patients, and staff felt a rise in energy and reported being refreshed and rejuvenated. Similarly, close to even proportions reported a cognitive shift (they had thought things over or had worked out a problem, etc.). There was a predictable difference between the rates within the user types who felt more relaxed or calmed down (a drop in energy level) (see Figure 10–3), and also be-

## FIGURE 10–1

### The Percentages of Each User Type Who Bring Their Children to Play in the Garden

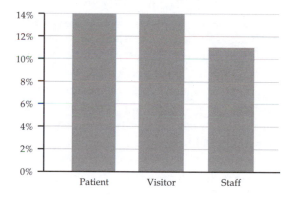

Bring Kids to Play Here

## FIGURE 10–2

### The Percentages of Each User Type Who Visit with (Other) Patients in the Garden

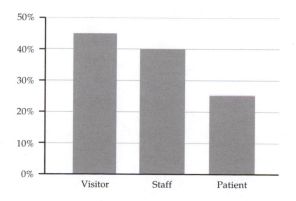

Visit with Patients

FIGURE 10–3

*The Percentages of Each User Type Who
Report a Pleasing Drop in Energy Level*

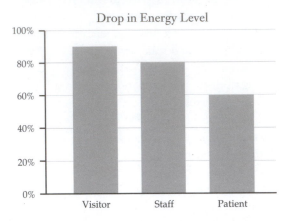

Drop in Energy Level

tween those who reported spiritual or religious experiences and feelings (see Figure 10–4).

The different user-patterns of these two mood shifts could be expected considering that patients are most probably physically ill, and the most likely users to be depressed or sad. It would follow, therefore, that they would seek an uplifting experience in the garden described by them as "religious" or "spiritual."

It was anticipated that some differences in responses would arise among the different sites. It was also expected that the length of time spent in the garden would be related to mood change. However, the analysis of the data did not support either of these assumptions. There were, however, differences in the proportion of user types at each site and these could be direct-

**FIGURE 10–4**

*The Percentages of Each User Type Who
Report a Spiritual or Religious Mood Shift*

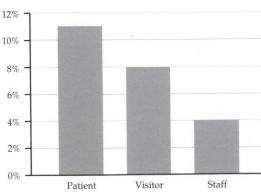

Deeper Meaning

ly associated with location and accessibility. At all of the sites except Alta Bates, about one-half of the interviewees were *employees*, with visitors and patients comprising the other half. In the roof garden at Alta Bates, however, more than 80 percent of the users were staff members. As discussed in chapter 7, this is a garden that is at one end of the hospital site, far from the main entry. The entire interior area of that floor has recently been converted to a secure unit, forcing most users to come and go from a single elevator at the end of the lengthy hallway that jogs its way through the various hospital additions. Volunteers at the information desk were unable to direct us there upon our first visit and it was not shown on any maps of the site. It is only visible from one set of patient rooms, on the fourth floor, so even to learn of its existence, one has to rely on an informal network of communication. The staff, with their longer tenure there and their relative ease of mobility, are the predominant users.

The split between the proportion of *visitor* and *patient* users was relatively even for Kaiser Walnut Creek and Alta Bates. There were substantial differences between these groups at San Francisco General, however, where many more patients were interviewed than visitors. At this site, the issue is not one of accessibility; rather it is one of location. The garden is directly outside two buildings that house several outpatient clinics that primarily serve adults (methadone maintenance, tuberculosis, HIV, family planning, etc.). The occasion for visitors to come here is much more limited than at a site adjacent to an inpatient building.

## In Summary

This research has documented that people in medical settings use available outdoor gardens for therapy and emotional healing. Positive perspectives and attitudes are known to support better health and increased recovery rates from illness. The beneficial emotional changes reported by patients after spending time in the garden, *and* being cared for by staff who have the opportunity to rejuvenate themselves and return to work more relaxed and refreshed, must then improve the healing environment. The increased morale of the employees contributes to the smooth functioning of a productive and efficient work force, increasing the level of satisfaction for the total hospital community.

Patients, visitors, and staff come to the garden to help themselves to feel better. They do this consciously, and speak eloquently about the gardens and their experiences there. They come to get away, to relax, and to think and build their strength. They report as significant:

• plants and growing, living things
• varied sensory stimulation
• facilitation of the psychological experience of expansiveness and peacefulness

• opportunities for social interaction and observation.

By examining these sites individually and in aggregate, issues of site planning, accessibility, and the need for a space that is in *contrast* with the controlled and sterile internal environment clearly come to the fore. In the following chapter, design recommendations are presented that arise from the discussions and interviews and the observations at both the case study sites and the sites presented in the typology chapter.

# 11. DESIGN RECOMMENDATIONS

THE FOLLOWING RECOMMENDATIONS have emerged from the case studies and from additional brief critical evaluations of outdoor spaces at other hospitals described in chapter 5. The recommendations are divided into three groups:

A) locational, site-planning, and way-finding;
B) planting, seating, aesthetic, and detail;
C) policy regarding the provision and maintenance of gardens intended to be used for therapeutic benefit.

## A. Locational, Site Planning, and Way-Finding Recommendations

To truly maximize the potential of garden spaces in hospital facilities, the design process needs to begin with site planning. Many issues that we encountered in our research could have been mitigated or avoided if the provision of potentially therapeutic garden spaces had been considered from the beginning. Accordingly, our recommendations start with a number of steps that are often overlooked.

Principles for site planning of therapeutic garden environments in healthcare facilities are:

- Healthcare facilities are high-stress environments for staff and patients alike. Exterior environments should provide a contrast to the interior space, in order to facilitate a sense of "getting away."
- Physically ill people are a vulnerable population. They are acutely aware of their physical

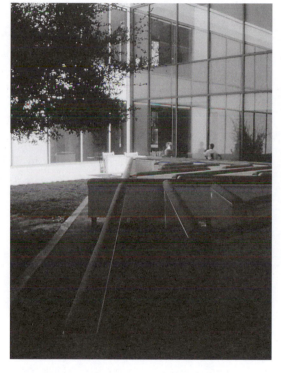

Photo 11–1: *Children enjoy this imaginative maze, lawn, and climbing tree in a courtyard adjacent to the pediatric department of this suburban medical center. Surrounded by plate-glass windows, this space allows easy monitoring, yet provides sound insulation for children who need to let off steam. (Kaiser Permanente Medical Center, Vallejo, CA)*

comfort. Design with particular awareness of issues of mobility and microclimate.

- People who are not well also tend to be emotionally vulnerable and sometimes intellectually impaired. Design for a sense of security, serenity, and safety — with defined seating areas, easily readable pathways, and clear designations — and remember the symbolic takes on increased meaning as we grapple with our own frailties.

Specific suggestions include:

1. A professional landscape architect needs to be on the design team from the start to as-

sist with the determination of outdoor space location, orientation, function, and ambience, and to assess microclimates, accessibility, and anticipated user groups.

2. Since there are likely to be multiple users (staff, inpatients, outpatients, visitors), with a range in ages, including children, the planning of a new hospital, or hospital addition, should include consideration of a variety of outdoor spaces. These need to be varied as to *type* (i.e., front porch, roof garden, courtyard, etc.) and design *image*: for example, an entry porch where people can sit and wait for a taxi; a terrace or courtyard off the cafeteria for outdoor eating; an attractive viewing garden where people waiting for appointments or for items at the pharmacy can sit and look out at greenery; a ground-level or roof garden that has the immediate imagery of "a garden," and which is furnished and detailed for quiet contemplation, eating a brown-bag lunch, meditation, strolling, and so on.

3. Our field studies revealed that lack of *knowledge* about the existence of a garden space is one of the most critical factors in its use. The location and visibility of such spaces is very important. One outdoor space should be visible from the main entrance or there should be clear and prominent directions as to its location.

4. The amount of time to spend outside is limited, especially for employees of a healthcare facility. A garden, courtyard, or roof terrace next to the cafeteria can draw people into the fresh air, offering a choice and allowing them to take best advantage of the free time. Also, in most hospitals now, this is the only space where one can eat and smoke.

Photo 11–2:
*A covered sitting terrace with forest views outside a day room offers convenient access to the outdoors in all weather, as well as visibility for monitoring by staff. Movable chairs provide a residential feeling while allowing for a variety of social groupings. (Monterey County Hospice, Monterey, CA)*

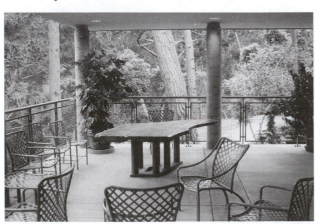

5. Outdoor spaces designed to optimize therapeutic benefits need to have a degree of enclosure or separation from the outside world — an entry lawn or landscaped setback from the street is not appropriate as the only space available for use.

6. Visibility of a garden space from inside for staff monitoring of patients is especially critical for long-term care facilities. Patio areas off day rooms are a successful combination.

7. Where there is sufficient room, divide the space so that there are sub-areas of varying size and levels of privacy. Some users come alone and seek a space in which to sit that is comfortably private, while others may desire distraction and social interaction.

8. The interior and exterior spaces should complement each other. If patients near an outdoor space have private rooms, exterior areas for social interaction and observation should be a priority. If nearby units have an open, multiple-bed floor plan, more areas for private conversations and withdrawing from social interaction need to be provided.

9. Balconies or roof terraces with a view into a garden can add to the use of an outdoor space, especially for those on gurneys or in wheelchairs who cannot easily access the garden proper. These spaces need to be of ample size and have wide doors — perhaps automatic — so that visitors and volunteers, who may not be experienced in moving patients, feel that the space is accessible, without having to worry about mobility.

10. The layout of the garden needs to be easily "readable," to minimize confusion for those who are not functioning well. This is especially true in nursing homes and facilities for patients with psychological impairment.

11. Make sure that the garden is easily accessible to patients and the paving surface is wide enough to accommodate wheelchairs and gurneys.

## B. Planting, Seating, and Detail Recommendations

In keeping with the main focus of this report, the following recommendations on design details and planting refer to garden spaces where patients, staff, etc., are likely to go to relax, to think and build their strength, and to get away from the hospital environment. Our interviews and case studies clearly indicate that three aspects of design details are critical in facilitating a change of mood and lowering stress. These are the presence of a variety of green, growing, and living things; the stimulation of the senses; and the availability of a variety of settings for both social interaction and quiet introspection.

The following design principles can serve as guides to creating therapeutic garden environments:

- Provide sensory stimuli that is noninvasive in character to draw our attention away from the initial feeling state to an external focus.
- Facilitate physical and psychological movement with pathways and/or vistas through to a variety of types of spaces, thereby assisting a shift in perspective.
- Create areas for safe seclusion as well as social interaction to help think and work through issues.

Specific suggestions to achieve these goals are:

1. Lush, colorful planting that is varied and eye-catching so as to suggest the image of a garden. Over and over, trees, plants, and greenery were cited as the most significant helpful characteristic.

2. Appropriate plant selection, with special attention given to cultural requirements and correct placement in the garden, is one of the essential elements of a therapeutic garden environment, as dying and unhealthy plants have a negative psychological impact on those observing them.

3. Flowering trees, shrubs, and perennials provide a sense of seasonal change that reinforces one's awareness of life's rhythms and cycles.

4. Trees whose foliage moves easily, even in a slight breeze, draw the user's attention to the patterns of color, shadows, light, and movement. This was described by interviewees as a soothing and meditative experience.

5. Features to attract birds — such as a fountain or birdbath, a bird feeder, trees appropriate for roosting or nesting — stimulate the senses and help to lift people's spirits.

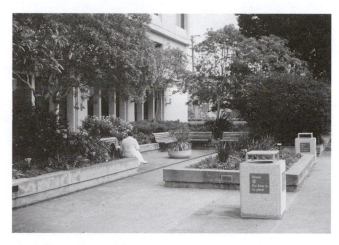

6. Contrast and harmony in texture, form, color, and arrangement of plant materials provide a variety that holds the attention and helps to draw our focus away from ourselves.

7. Plant species that attract butterflies call attention to the ephemeral, serving as a gentle reminder of the preciousness of life.

8. In addition to providing an external focus, sound can create a psychological screen (white noise) that serves the restoration process. A water feature can provide this pleasing and soothing sound. Care should be taken to place it in a wind-protected location where people can sit nearby, and where air-conditioning or other irritating noises do not create too much competition.

9. For the comfort of users, where offices or patient rooms border the garden, create a planting buffer of sufficient distance and depth so that people walking or sitting in the garden do not feel that they are intruding on the privacy of those indoors.

10. Paths that meander allow for strolling and contemplation and complement more heavily used direct routes between access points. Where the space is large enough, provide varying vistas, levels of shade, and textures of planting along these routes.

11. Select paving surfaces that are smooth enough to accommodate wheelchairs and gurneys.

12. In long-term facilities, arrange entrances to the garden and width of pathways so that volunteers or family members can easily bring a patient on a gurney or in a wheelchair out into the space.

Photo 11–3:
*This roof terrace in a larger urban hospital offers a promenade for strolling (to the right of photo) and semiprivate seating clusters incorporating the warm textural materials of brick and wood. The terrace offers sun or shade, and views toward greenery or over the city skyline. (St. Mary's Hospital, San Francisco, CA)*

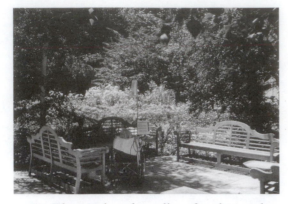

13. Electrical outlets allow for the garden to be used for hospital parties or other spon-sored functions, extending the use to other people who may not usually come.

14. Nighttime lighting maximizes the ther-apeutic benefit by allowing people to use the space safely after dark, or to look out at the garden from indoors.

15. Seating arranged for social interaction (right angled or centripetal benches, or mov-able chairs) near to the entrance into the gar-den adds convenience, as this area will likely be used for quick smoking breaks by staff who know each other.

16. Seating partly enclosed by planting, or at the perimeter of an open space, provides a degree of privacy for those wanting to be alone, or who want to observe from a distance.

17. Fixed seating with backs for sitting in comfort is especially important for garden users who may be physically weak.

18. If bench-type seating is provided, select a material that is appealing to the touch (i.e., wood) and a size (4–6 feet) such that one or two people can "claim" the space. The image might be of a garden bench, rather than a park or bus stop bench.

19. Increase the seating options available with movable seating so that users can meet their own particular needs. These chairs can be moved, selecting the degree of sun and shade, as well as determining the size of the seating cluster.

20. Benches, platform seating, or planter-edge seating with something to support the back allows people to sit with their feet up — or they can lie down to take a nap or sunbathe, as was frequently observed.

21. Tables with movable chairs or benches provide for users who want to hold a meeting

or eat, especially where the space is adjacent to the cafeteria.

22. Adjustable umbrellas allow people to control the amount of sun or shade, so impor-tant to those who feel unwell or are taking cer-tain medications.

23. Wind shelters, heat-reflecting surfaces — or alternatively, shade-producing arbors — and other structures and planting help to miti-gate the climate, and extend the use of the gar-den into several seasons.

24. Where there is a view, make sure that some seating faces that direction to facilitate psychological movement out of the space. If the exterior space is a roof garden or terrace, the edge rail, balustrade, or planter should be sufficiently low or transparent so that people seated can take in the view.

25. Where there is not a ready-made view, a sense of mystery and movement can be cre-ated by designing smaller-scale glimpses and intriguing focal points within the garden, to draw the users' attention and, sometimes, fa-cilitate a change in perspective.

26. Providing one or more eye-catching and unique features by which people will iden-

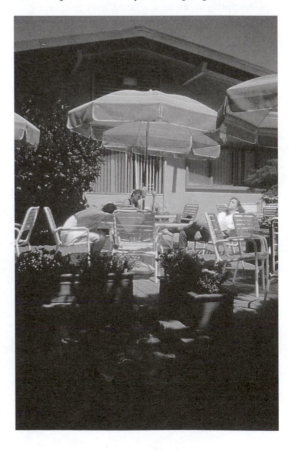

tify a garden — such as a sculpture, wind chimes, an aviary, a fish pond — serves to anchor memories of the garden and the restoration achieved there.

## C. Policy and Maintenance recommendations

One of the interesting contrasts that we discovered during our canvassing of potential research sites was that we encountered what appeared to be more emphasis on the garden spaces and a greater awareness of potential therapeutic benefits at the public institutions than at private facilities. The older public facilities take great pride in their gardens, and there was a high level of awareness of their place in the healing milieu of the facility. Private institutions, on the other hand, appear to view incorporated gardens primarily as cosmetic elements. Older established gardens in these private hospitals have gone to seed, or have been encroached upon. Decisions made by the hospital administration do have a direct impact on the success of exterior therapeutic garden spaces. These are the principles and guidelines that we recommend.

- Exterior garden spaces are a resource to be used for maximum benefit; promoting awareness and facilitating use will influence the level of benefit derived.
- Considering a garden as an essential element within the therapeutic milieu of a facility gives additional variation and support to the entire hospital community.
- Quality maintenance contributes to the health of the plants, which in turn provides the maximum therapeutic benefit.

Specific recommendations:

1. Our field studies revealed that awareness of the garden space is one of the most critical factors in its use. We found that even where there was an outdoor space, people at the information desk were often not aware of its existence, or mistaken about accessibility. (The extreme situation was in one hospital where it took 45 minutes and several exasperating trails of misinformation before access could be attained to a locked roof garden that was "open to the public.") Signs that direct people

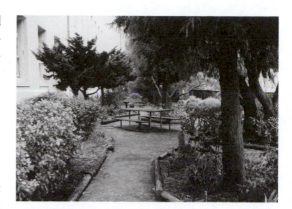

to the space, labeling the gardens on posted maps, and listing them in the resource handbook at the information desk would go a long way toward promoting their use and reaping their rewards.

2. Educating employees about the existence and therapeutic benefits of exterior spaces will increase their use of the gardens and contribute toward a refreshed, rejuvenated, and more productive staff.

3. Encouraging the medical staff to promote the use of exterior spaces will increase the use of gardens by patients and visitors, and extend the ripple of the beneficial effect to everyone.

4. Scheduling events and meetings in the garden incorporates the restorative benefits of a garden into the work schedule.

5. Communication can be easier in an exterior space. Several interviewees mentioned that the gardeners provided companionship and were great to talk to. The head gardener at one of the study sites remarked on the public relations service he provided, by listening to people vent and express their dissatisfactions. The casual nature of being in the garden can enhance communication; acknowledging this and capitalizing on it would benefit the entire organization.

6. Keep gardens open; appealing gardens, designed with seating but that are behind locked doors, are as bad or worse than nothing. The frustration that rattling locked doors creates increases the stress levels of newcomers to the facility (and the emotional cost would be even greater, and longer term, to those who may be confused or disoriented). Gardens that are designed for use should be kept available.

7. In a time when money is limited, creative thinking can lead to increased benefit. Recruitment and use of volunteers to take patients outside gives relief to the staff as well as to the patients.

8. Consider approaching volunteers or a local garden club to raise money for, and/or to maintain, a hospital garden.

9. Maintenance is important in terms of both the physical safety of the site and the therapeutic potential. Shrubs, trees, and flowers are labor intensive compared to structures and patio spaces. Yet it is these green, growing things that appear to offer the most restorative value. Appropriate fertilizing, selective thinning rather than shearing, and the use of seasonal color contribute to the healthy and natural qualities listed as significant by the users of the study.

10. Encouraging birds, butterflies, squirrels, etc. — another aspect of the garden that is high on the list of significant qualities — is easier if organic practices are employed. Undocumented but also relevant may be the detrimental effect of the use of chemicals on the health of the people in the garden, especially those who are already physically unwell. Hand weeding, mulching, companion planting, and appropriate spacing of plants all reduce the need for the use of chemicals.

11. Interest, variety, the fact that "someone cares" about the garden were mentioned by users of the garden; pristine lines, perfection, and aesthetic excellence were not. Maintenance should be geared toward providing a friendly, comfortable, welcoming space rather than perfection.

# 12. CONCLUSION

**T**HIS STUDY HAS explored the use of hospital gardens and the therapeutic benefits of these outdoor spaces. By observing and interviewing people while they are in the garden, the benefits of these spaces have been described and documented. Ninety-five percent of the people in the gardens reported a therapeutic benefit. Employees said they were more productive, patients spoke of feeling better and having more tolerance for their medical procedures, and friends and relatives felt relief from the stress of the hospital visit.

Some important questions arise from this study: Is there documentation for increasing the amount of common area outside? What, if any, are the differences in the design of gardens for different patient populations? What are the comments from people who do not use a garden, when there is one available and accessible? Why don't they use it? Is it a question of personal preference?

The next step in the pursuit of full utilization of all space in healthcare facilities is to compare the results of this study with a similar one examining interior spaces. What are the therapeutic benefits of common areas such as day rooms, waiting rooms, and cafeterias? And are there any design elements mentioned in this research on gardens that can be applied to interior spaces?

There is no question of the perceived therapeutic benefits of the garden spaces reported in this research. Narrowing the scope of subsequent research to accommodate specific quantitative analysis and conducting comparative studies to establish the place of the garden on the fiscal priority list of healthcare facilities are challenges that lie ahead.

# APPENDIX
## *Questionnaire*

**Location**

_____

_____

_____

**Date and Time** _____

**Number** _____

1) The oral consent script has been read and consent given?

❏ yes
❏ no

2) Gender is:

❏ female
❏ male

3) Would you mind telling me if you are:

❏ employee
❏ patient who is in the hospital
❏ outpatient here for a doctor appointment, test, shot, etc.
❏ visitor

4) How often do you come out here?

❏ my first time
❏ occasionally, sometimes
❏ once or twice a week
❏ every day
❏ several times a day

5) What do you generally do out here? *(several boxes may be checked)*

❏ sit and wait (for an appointment, a friend, etc.)
❏ sit and relax (smoke, read, have coffee, etc.)
❏ sit and talk with friend(s), colleague(s)
❏ hold a work-related meeting
❏ visit with a patient (sit, stroll, etc.)
❏ walk through on my way to another building
❏ come out for a stroll (not necessarily en route to another building)
❏ let my kids run and play here
❏ outdoor therapy
❏ eat
❏ other _____

6) When you come out here, how long do you generally stay? *(may give several answers, depending on activity)*

❏ just a few minutes
❏ 5–10 minutes
❏ 10–30 minutes
❏ more than 30 minutes

7) Is there anything that prevents or inhibits you from coming here as much as you would like?

8) What do you like best about this place?

9) Is there anything you would like to see changed or added?

11) What specific characteristics or qualities of this place help you to feel _____?
*(fill in the answer to question 10)*

10) Do you feel any different after you've spent time in the garden?

12) Is there anything else you would like to tell me about the garden, or how you feel when you are out here?

# BIBLIOGRAPHY

Barnes, Marni. "Emotional Healing in the Wilderness and Its Implications for the Built Environment." Unpublished paper, Berkeley, CA, 1993.

Barnes, Marni. "A Study of the Process of Emotional Healing in Outdoor Spaces and the Concomitant Landscape Design Implications." MLA thesis, Department of Landscape Architecture, University of California, Berkeley, 1994.

Carpman, J.R., M.A. Grant, and D.A. Simmons, *Design that Cares: Planning Health Facilities for Patients and Visitors.* Chicago: American Hospital Association, 1986.

Chambers, Nancy. "Therapeutic Horticulture Gardens." *Journal of Healthcare Design*, Vol. VII, pp. 169–174.

Delaney, Christopher, and James Burnett. "Design Quality: Landscape Design — Improving the Quality of Health Care." *Journal of Healthcare Design*, Vol. VI, pp. 153–162.

Ewert, Alan. "Reducing Levels of Trait Anxiety Through the Application of Wilderness-based Activities." *The Use of Wilderness for Personal Growth Therapy and Education.* General Technical Report RM 193, pp. 105–111. Ft. Collins, CO: United States Forest Service, 1990.

Francis, Carolyn, and Claire Cooper Marcus. "Places People Take Their Problems." *Proceedings of the 22nd Annual Conference of the Environmental Design Research Association.* Mexico, 1991.

Francis, Carolyn, and Claire Cooper Marcus. "Restorative Places: Environment and Emotional Well-being." Unpublished paper, Berkeley, CA, 1992.

Francis, Mark, P. Lindsay, and Jay Rice (eds.). The *Healing Dimensions of People-Plant Relations: Conference Proceedings.* Center for Design Research, University of California, Davis, 1994.

Gibson, Peter M. "Therapeutic Aspects of Wilderness Programs: A Comprehensive Literature Review." *Therapeutic Recreational Journal*, second quarter, 1979. Arlington, VA: National Therapeutic Recreation Society.

Greenway, Robert. "An Eighteen-Year Investigation of 'Wilderness Therapy.'" *The Use of Wilderness for Personal Growth Therapy and Education.* General Technical Report RM 193, pp. 103–104. Ft. Collins, CO: United States Forest Service, 1990.

_____. "Mapping the Wilderness Experience: ideas and questions gleaned from an 18-year study of a University Wilderness Program." Unpublished manuscript, Rohnert Park, CA, 1989.

Hartig, Terry, et al. "Perspectives on Wilderness: Testing the Theory of Restorative Environments." *The Use of Wilderness for Personal Growth Therapy and Education.* General Technical Report RM 193, pp. 86–95. Ft. Collins, CO: United States Forest Service, 1990.

Healy, Vince. "The Hospice Garden: The Visitor and the Grieving Process." Unpublished paper presented at The Meanings of the Garden Conference. Davis, CA, 1991.

_____. "The Hospice Garden: Addressing the Patient's Needs Through Landscape." Unpublished paper, San Francisco, CA, 1994.

Honeyman, M. "Vegetation and Stress: A comparison study of varying amounts of vegetation in countryside and urban scenes." MLA thesis, Department of Landscape Architecture, Kansas State University, Manhattan, KS, 1987.

Kaplan, Rachel. "Some Psychological Benefits of Gardening." *Environment and Behavior*, 1973, pp. 145–61.

Kaplan, Stephen, and Janet Talbot. "Psychological Benefits of a Wilderness Experience." In *Behavior and the Natural Environment*, edited by I. Altman and J.F. Wohlwil, 163–203. New York: Plenum, 1983.

Kimball, Richard. "The Wilderness as Therapy," *Journal of Experiential Education* 3 (1983): 6–9.

Minter, Sue. *The Healing Garden*. London: Headline Book Publishing, 1994.

Mooney, Patrick. "Gardens as a Prosthetic Tool: The Garden Design of a Residential Facility for Alzheimer's Patients." Unpublished paper presented at the Healing Aspects of People-Plant Relations Symposium, Davis, CA, 1994.

Paine, Robert, and Carolyn Francis. "Hospital Outdoor Spaces." In *People Places: Design Guidelines for Urban Open Space*, edited by Clare Cooper Marcus and Carolyn Francis, *263*–288. New York: Van Nostrand Reinhold, 1990.

Russell, James, and Jacalyn Snodgrass. "Emotion and the Environment." In *Handbook of Environmental Psychology: Vol. I*, edited by Daniel Stokols and Irwin Altman. 1987.

Stainbrook, E. "Human Needs and the Natural Environment." *Man and Nature in the City Symposium*, 1–6. Washington, DC: Bureau of Sport Fisheries and Wildlife, U.S. Department of the Interior, 1968.

Thompson, John, and Grace Golden. *The Hospital: A Social and Architectural History*. New Haven, CT: Yale University Press.

Ulrich, Roger. "Visual Landscapes and Psychological Well-Being." *Landscape Research* 4 (1979): 17–23.
———. "View Through a Window May Influence Recovery from Surgery." *Science* No: 224 (1984): 420–421.

———. "The Psychological Benefits of Plants." *Garden*, November/December (1984).

———. "Human Responses to Vegetation and Landscapes." *Landscape and Planning* 13 (1986): 29–44.

———. "Aesthetic and Affective Responses to Natural Environments." In *Human Behavior and Environment, Vol. 6*, edited by I. Altman and J.F. Wohlwil, 85–125. New York: Plenum Press,

Ulrich, Roger, and R. Parsons. "Influences of Passive Experiences with Plants on Individual Well-Being and Social Development." Unpublished paper presented at the National Symposium of the Role of Horticulture on Human Well-Being and Social Development. Washington, DC, April 19–21, 1990.

Ulrich, Roger, and R.F. Simons. "Recovery from Stress During Exposure to Everyday Outdoor Environments." *Proceedings of the 17th Annual Conference of the Environmental Design Research Association*, 115–22. Washington, DC, 1989.

Warner, Sam Bass Jr. "Restorative Gardens: Recovering Some Human Wisdom for Modern Design." Unpublished paper, 1995.